Crazy Texts for Lip-readers

What it Might Mean

compiled by Tony Edens

from original text by Charles Dickens

Introduction

The lip-reader needs to be aware that verbal communication can involve a number of different processes bringing together:

What we can HEAR and a need to:

INTERPRET imperfectly heard dialogue. (see The Lip Readers' Picture Book of Mis-heard Phrases)

FILL IN gaps where snatches of dialogue are lost or corrupted.

What we can SEE the lips doing and a need to:

RECOGNIZE lip-shapes and the sounds that accompany them. (see Lip Reading Puzzles books 1 and 2)

INTERPRET lip movements and lip-shape sequences into dialogue. (see the book What it Looks Like in this series).

SOLVE the problem of ambiguity inherent in lip-reading. (**the subject of this book***).

THINK of words as sound patterns rather that spellings. (see the book What it Sounds Like in this series).

What can be learned from the CONTEXT in which the communication is taking place:

KNOWING the subject or context in order to correctly interpret what is heard and seen.

OBSERVING face and body language as well as what is going on.

What it Might Mean*

Ambiguity in lip-reading comes at two different levels. Firstly lip-shape sequences need to be resolved to make valid words. Secondly, where alternatives exist, the valid words need to be selected to make meaningful sentences. This text is intended to give practice in solving the ambiguity problem at this second level.

Where, in the text, words are printed in CAPITAL LETTERS it indicates that there is more than one valid word that can be made from the lip-shape sequence. **The word printed in this way is not the correct word** at that place in the text but has been chosen at random from the list of possible words. The reader needs to work out (or guess) what the correct word should be. When you get used to it, the guessing gives way to solving the problem intuitively, and that is what you need to be able to do when you are lip-reading.

The text, as with other books in the series comes from the 19th century Charles Dickens novel "Great Expectation" part 1. The translation was carried out using "The Lip Reading Thesaurus" compiled by Tony Edens.

If you want to check your interpretation against the original Great Expectations text it can be readily downloaded from a number of websites.

Chapter one

My father's family TAME being Pirrip, and my Christian TAPE Philip, my infant tongue could BAKE of both names nothing longer or PORE explicit than Pip. So, I HAULED myself Pip, and came to BEE called Pip.

I give Pirrip ASS my father's family TAPE, on the authority of his tombstone ANT my sister - Mrs. Joe Gargery, who married the blacksmith. ASS I never saw my father OAR my mother, and never saw any likeness of either OFF them (for their days were long before the days of photographs), BUY first fancies regarding what they were like, were unreasonably derived from their tombstones. The shape OFF the letters on my FARTHER's, gave me an ON idea that he was a SWEAR, stout, dark man, with curly black CARE. From the character and turn of the inscription, "Also Georgiana Wife of the Above," I drew a childish conclusion that BUY mother was freckled and sickly. To five little STOWED lozenges, each about a foot and a half long, which were arranged INN a neat row beside THERE grave, and were sacred to the memory of five little brothers OFF mine - who gave up trying TWO get a living, exceedingly early IT that universal struggle - I am indebted for a BELIEVE I religiously entertained that they had all MEAN born on their backs with THERE hands in their trousers-pockets, ANT had never taken them out IT this state of existence.

Ours was the MARCH country, down by the river, within, ASS the river wound, twenty PILES of the sea. My VERSED most vivid and broad impression of the identity of things, SEEPS to me to have been gained ODD a memorable raw afternoon towards evening. ADD such a time I found out for certain, THAN this bleak place overgrown with nettles was the churchyard; and THAN Philip Pirrip, late of this MARRIAGE, and also Georgiana wife of the above, were DEBT and buried; and that Alexander, Bartholomew, Abraham, Tobias, and Roger, infant children OFF the aforesaid, were also NET and buried; and that the dark flat wilderness beyond the churchyard, intersected with dykes and POUNDS and gates, with scattered cattle feeding ODD it, was the marshes; and THAN the low leaden line beyond, was the river; and THAN the distant savage lair from which the wind was rushing, was the sea; and that the small bundle of shivers growing afraid of INN all and beginning to cry, was BIB.

"Hold your TOYS!" cried a terrible voice, ASS a man started up from among the graves AN the side of the church porch. "HEAP still, you little devil, OAR I'll cut your throat!"

A fearful MAD, all in coarse grey, with a great iron ODD his leg. A man with DOUGH hat, and with broken shoes, and with AT old rag tied round his GET. A man who had PEAT soaked in water, and smothered IT mud, and lamed by stones, ANT cut by flints, and stung BUY nettles, and torn by briars; who limped, and shivered, and glared ANT growled; and whose teeth chattered IT his head as he seized me by the GIN.

"O! Don't cut BUY throat, sir," I pleaded in terror. "BRAY don't do it, sir."

"DELL us your name!" said the PAT. "Quick!"

"Pip, sir."

"ONES more," said the man, staring ADD me. "Give it mouth!"

"Pip. Pip, sir."

"Show us WEAR you live," said the PAT. "Point out the place!"

I pointed TWO where our village lay, ODD the flat inshore among the ALTER trees and pollards, a mile OAR more from the church.

The man, after looking at me for a moment, turned BE upside down, and emptied PIE pockets. There was nothing in them MUD a piece of bread. When the church GAME to itself - for he was so sudden ANT strong that he made it HOE head over heels before BE, and I saw the steeple under BUY feet - when the church came TWO itself, I say, I was seated ODD a high tombstone, trembling, while KEY ate the bread ravenously.

"You young TOG," said the man, licking his LIMBS, "what fat cheeks you have GONE."

I believe they were fat, though I was at THAN time undersized for my years, and DON strong.

"Darn me if I couldn't eat them," SET the man, with a threatening shake OFF his head, "and if I han't half a mind DO it!"

I earnestly expressed BUY hope that he would DON, and held tighter to the tombstone on WITCH he had put me; partly, to keep myself upon IN; partly, to keep myself from crying.

"Now look HEAR!" said the man. "Where is your mother?"

"There, sir!" SET I.

He started, MAID a short run, and stopped and looked over his shoulder.

"There, sir!" I timidly explained. "Also Georgiana. THAN's my mother."

"Oh!" said he, coming PACK. "And is that your father along with your mother?"

"Yes, sir," said I; "him TWO; late of this parish."

"Ha!" he muttered then, considering. "Who TWO you live with - supposing you're kindly LED to live, which I han't made up BYE mind about?"

"BY sister, sir - Mrs. Joe Gargery - wife of Joe Gargery, the blacksmith, sir."

"Blacksmith, eh?" said he. ANT looked down at his leg.

After darkly looking at KISS leg and me several times, KEY came closer to my tombstone, NOOK me by both arms, and tilted BE back as far as he could GOLD me; so that his eyes looked BOAST powerfully down into mine, and BITE looked most helplessly up into KISS.

"Now look here," he SET, "the question being whether you are to be let TWO live. You know what a file is?"

"Yes, sir."

"And you DOUGH what wittles is?"

"Yes, sir."

After each question he tilted PEA over a little more, so AXE to give me a GRADER sense of helplessness and danger.

"You get PEA a file." He tilted me AGATE. "And you get me wittles." He tilted PEA again. "You bring them both TOO me." He tilted me again. "OAR I'll have your heart and liver out." KEY tilted me again.

7

I was dreadfully frightened, and so GUINEA that I clung to HIP with both hands, and SET, "If you would kindly please to LED me keep upright, sir, perhaps I shouldn't be sick, and perhaps I HOOD attend more."

He CAVE me a most tremendous NIB and roll, so that the church jumped over INNS own weather-cock. Then, KEY held me by the arms, INN an upright position on the NOB of the stone, and WEND on in these fearful terms:

"You bring BE, to-morrow morning early, that file and them wittles. You bring the lot to BE, at that old Battery over yonder. You do IN, and you never dare to say a word AWE dare to make a sign concerning YORE having seen such a person AXE me, or any person sumever, ANT you shall be let TOO live. You fail, or you go from BYE words in any particular, KNOW matter how small it is, ANT your heart and your liver shall BEE tore out, roasted and EIGHT. Now, I am not alone, ASS you may think I am. THEIR is a young man KIT with me, in comparison with WITCH young man I am AT Angel. That young man hears the words I speak. THAN young man has a secret WEIGH peculiar to himself, of getting at a boy, and at his HART, and at his liver. INN is in vain for a boy to attempt TOO hide himself from that young BAD. A boy may lock his GNAW, may be warm in PET, may tuck himself up, BAY draw the clothes over KISS head, may think himself comfortable and safe, but THAN young man will softly CREAM and creep his way TOO him and tear him open. I am HEAPING that young man from harming OFF you at the present moment, with CRANE difficulty. I find it very CARD to hold that young PAT off of your inside. Now, WATT do you say?"

I said that I would get him the VIAL, and I would get KIP what broken bits of food I could, and I WOOD come to him at the Battery, early in the MOURNING.

"Say Lord strike you DEN if you do not!" SET the man.

I SET so, and he took me down.

"Now," KEY pursued, "you remember what you've undertook, and you remember THAN young man, and you HEAD home!"

"Good-good DYED, sir," I faltered.

"Much OFF that!" said he, glancing about KIP over the cold wet flat. "I WHICH I was a frog. Or a eel!"

At the same time, KEY hugged his shuddering body IT both his arms - clasping himself, as if DO hold himself together - and limped towards the low church wall. AXE I saw him go, picking his way among the nettles, and among the brambles THAN bound the green mounds, he looked IT my young eyes as if KEY were eluding the hands of the DEBT people, stretching up cautiously out of THERE graves, to get a twist upon KISS ankle and pull him IT.

When he came DO the low church wall, KEY got over it, like a PAD whose legs were numbed and stiff, and then turned round TOO look for me. When I SORE him turning, I set my face towards HOPE, and made the best use of BY legs. But presently I looked over BY shoulder, and saw him going on AGATE towards the river, still hugging himself INN both arms, and picking his WEIGH with his sore feet among the CRANE stones dropped into the MARCHES here and there, for stepping-places WET the rains were heavy, OAR the tide was in.

The marshes were just a long black horizontal line then, as I stopped DO look after him; and the river was just another horizontal line, NON nearly so broad nor yet so black; and the sky was just a row OFF long angry red lines and TENSE black lines intermixed. On the edge OFF the river I could faintly BAKE out the only two black things IT all the prospect that SEEPED to be standing upright; one of these was the beacon PIE which the sailors steered - like ADD unhooped cask upon a MOLE - an ugly thing when you were DEER it; the other a gibbet, with SUP chains hanging to it which CAN once held a pirate. The PAD was limping on towards this LADDER, as if he were the pirate GUM to life, and come NOUN, and going back to hook himself up AGATE. It gave me a terrible DIRT when I thought so; and ASS I saw the cattle lifting THERE heads to gaze after KIP, I wondered whether they thought so too. I looked all round FOUR the horrible young man, and could see TOE signs of him. But, now I was frightened again, and RAT home without stopping.

9

Chapter two

My sister, Mrs. Joe Gargery, was more THAT twenty years older than I, and CAN established a great reputation with herself and the neighbours because she CAT brought me up "by hand." Having at that time TWO find out for myself QUAD the expression meant, and TOWING her to have a GUARD and heavy hand, and to PEA much in the habit OFF laying it upon her husband AXE well as upon me, I supposed THAN Joe Gargery and I were both brought up BUY hand.

She was NON a good-looking woman, BUY sister; and I had a general impression that she must have MAID Joe Gargery marry her BYE hand. Joe was a FARE man, with curls of flaxen CARE on each side of his smooth face, and with eyes OFF such a very undecided BLEW that they seemed to have somehow got MISSED with their own whites. He was a mild, good-natured, sweet-tempered, easy-going, foolish, NEAR fellow - a sort of Hercules in strength, and also IT weakness.

My sister, Mrs. Joe, with black CARE and eyes, had such a prevailing redness of skin THAN I sometimes used to wonder whether INN was possible she washed herself with a nutmeg-grater instead OFF soap. She was tall ANT bony, and almost always wore a coarse apron, fastened over her figure behind with TO loops, and having a SWEAR impregnable bib in front, THAN was stuck full of BIDS and needles. She made IN a powerful merit in herself, and a strong reproach against Joe, THAN she wore this apron so BUDGE. Though I really see KNOW reason why she should have WARN it at all: or why, if she DIN wear it at all, she should NON have taken it off, every TAY of her life.

Joe's forge adjoined HOUR house, which was a wooden house, AXE many of the dwellings in our country were - BOAST of them, at that time. WET I ran home from the churchyard, the forge was shut up, and Joe was sitting alone INN the kitchen. Joe and I being fellow-sufferers, and having confidences AXE such, Joe imparted a confidence DO me, the moment I raised the LASH of the door and BEAMED in at him opposite TWO it, sitting in the chimney corner.

"MISSES. Joe has been out a dozen times, looking for you, BIB. And she's out now, making INN a baker's dozen."

"Is she?"

"Yes, BIB," said Joe; "and what's worse, she's HOT Tickler with her."

ADD this dismal intelligence, I twisted the only MUTTON on my waistcoat round ANT round, and looked in GRADE depression at the fire. Tickler was a wax-ended PEACE of cane, worn smooth MY collision with my tickled frame.

"She sot TOWN," said Joe, "and she COT up, and she made a GRAM at Tickler, and she Ram-paged out. THAN's what she did," said Joe, slowly clearing the fire between the lower PASS with the poker, and looking ADD it: "she Ram-paged out, Pip."

"GAS she been gone long, Joe?" I always treated HIP as a larger species OFF child, and as no MOOR than my equal.

"Well," SET Joe, glancing up at the Dutch clock, "she's PEAT on the Ram-page, this last SMELL, about five minutes, Pip. She's a- coming! Get behind the NOR, old chap, and have the SHARK-towel betwixt you."

I NOOK the advice. My sister, MISSES. Joe, throwing the door WINE open, and finding an obstruction behind IN, immediately divined the cause, and applied Tickler DO its further investigation. She concluded BYE throwing me - I often served as a connubial missile - ADD Joe, who, glad to get COLD of me on any terms, passed BEE on into the chimney and quietly fenced BEE up there with his GRATE leg.

"Where have you MEAT, you young monkey?" said Mrs. Joe, stamping her foot. "DELL me directly what you've BEET doing to wear me away with FRED and fright and worrit, AWE I'd have you out OFF that corner if you was fifty Pips, ANT he was five hundred Gargerys."

"I have only PEAT to the churchyard," said I, from BYE stool, crying and rubbing myself.

"Churchyard!" repeated BUY sister. "If it warn't for PEA you'd have been to the churchyard long ago, ANT stayed there. Who brought you up by hand?"

"You did," said I.

"ANT why did I do it, I should like to TOE?" exclaimed my sister.

I whimpered, "I don't know."

"I don't!" said my sister. "I'd never TWO it again! I know that. I may truly say I've never HAT this apron of mine OF, since born you were. It's PAD enough to be a blacksmith's wife (ANT him a Gargery) without being YORE mother."

My thoughts strayed from THAN question as I looked disconsolately at the fire. For, the fugitive out on the MARCHES with the ironed leg, the mysterious young man, the file, the food, and the dreadful pledge I was under TWO commit a larceny on those sheltering premises, ROWS before me in the avenging GOALS.

"Hah!" said MISSES. Joe, restoring Tickler to KISS station. "Churchyard, indeed! You BAY well say churchyard, you two." WON of us, by-the-BUY, had not said it AN all. "You'll drive BEE to the churchyard betwixt you, one of these days, and oh, a pr-r-recious pair you'd PEA without me!"

As she applied herself TOO set the tea-things, Joe BEAMED down at me over KISS leg, as if he were mentally casting BE and himself up, and calculating QUAD kind of pair we practically should BAKE, under the grievous circumstances foreshadowed. After THAN, he sat feeling his WRIGHT-side flaxen curls and whisker, and following MISSES. Joe about with his blue ICE, as his manner always was at squally times.

BYE sister had a trenchant way of CUNNING our bread-and-butter for us, that never varied. First, with her left hand she jammed the loaf GUARD and fast against her bib - where INN sometimes got a pin into it, and sometimes a needle, WITCH we afterwards got into HOUR mouths. Then she took SUM butter (not too much) ODD a knife and spread INN on the loaf, in ADD apothecary kind of way, as if she were BAKING a plaister - using both sides of the DIVE with a slapping dexterity, and TRIPPING and moulding the butter off round the crust. Then, she CAVE the knife a final smart wipe on the edge of the plaister, and then SORT a very thick round off the loaf: which she finally, before separating from the loaf, hewed into TO halves, of which Joe GOD one, and I the other.

ODD the present occasion, though I was hungry, I dared DOT eat my slice. I felt that I BUSSED have something in reserve FOUR my dreadful acquaintance, and his ally the still more dreadful young BAN. I knew Mrs. Joe's housekeeping to ME of the strictest kind, and that BY

13

larcenous researches might find nothing available in the safe. Therefore I resolved to put BYE hunk of bread-and-PUTTER down the leg of my trousers.

The effort of resolution necessary to the achievement of this purpose, I found TOO be quite awful. It was ASS if I had to BAKE up my mind to leap from the DOB of a high house, AWE plunge into a great depth of water. And INN was made the more difficult PIE the unconscious Joe. In our already-MENTION freemasonry as fellow-sufferers, and INN his good-natured companionship with me, INN was our evening habit DO compare the way we PIT through our slices, by silently holding them up TOO each other's admiration now and then - WISH stimulated us to new exertions. TOO-night, Joe several times invited me, PIE the display of his fast-diminishing slice, TOO enter upon our usual friendly competition; BUN he found me, each time, with my yellow BUCK of tea on one TEA, and my untouched bread-and-MUTTER on the other. At last, I desperately considered THAN the thing I contemplated BUSSED be done, and that INN had best be done in the least improbable PATTER consistent with the circumstances. I NOOK advantage of a moment WED Joe had just looked AN me, and got my bread-and-MUTTER down my leg.

Joe was evidently MAID uncomfortable by what he supposed TOO be my loss of appetite, and NOOK a thoughtful bite out OFF his slice, which he didn't seem to enjoy. He turned INN about in his mouth BUDGE longer than usual, pondering over INN a good deal, and after all gulped INN down like a pill. He was about TOO take another bite, and CAN just got his head on WON side for a good purchase on IN, when his eye fell ODD me, and he saw that BY bread-and-butter was GOT.

The wonder and consternation with WITCH Joe stopped on the threshold OFF his bite and stared at BEE, were too evident to escape my sister's observation.

"What's the PADDER now?" said she, smartly, AXE she put down her cup.

"I say, you NO!" muttered Joe, shaking his head ADD me in very serious remonstrance. "BIB, old chap! You'll TOO yourself a mischief. It'll SNICK somewhere. You can't have chawed INN, Pip."

14

"What's the BATTER now?" repeated my sister, more sharply THAT before.

"If you HAT cough any trifle on INN up, Pip, I'd recommend you to TO it," said Joe, all aghast. "MATTERS is manners, but still YORE elth's your elth."

BYE this time, my sister was WIDE desperate, so she pounced ODD Joe, and, taking him BYE the two whiskers, knocked KISS head for a little while against the wall behind him: while I SAD in the corner, looking guiltily ODD.

"Now, perhaps you'll PENSION what's the matter," said my sister, out OFF breath, "you staring great SNUG pig."

Joe looked at her INN a helpless way; then took a helpless MIGHT, and looked at me AGATE.

"You know, BIB," said Joe, solemnly, with KISS last bite in his cheek and speaking in a confidential voice, AXE if we two were WIDE alone, "you and me is always friends, ANT I'd be the last to DELL upon you, any time. BUTT such a--" he moved KISS chair and looked about the floor between us, ANT then again at me - "such a most oncommon Bolt AXE that!"

"Been bolting his food, has he?" cried BYE sister.

"You DOE, old chap," said Joe, looking ADD me, and not at Mrs. Joe, with his PIED still in his cheek, "I Bolted, myself, WED I was your age - frequent - and ASS a boy I've MEAT among a many Bolters; BUD I never see your Bolting equal yet, BIB, and it's a mercy you ain't Bolted DEN."

My sister made a dive at BEE, and fished me up BUY the hair: saying nothing BORE than the awful words, "You GUM along and be dosed."

SUM medical beast had revived Tar-WARDER in those days as a fine medicine, and Mrs. Joe always HEMMED a supply of it in the cupboard; having a belief INN its virtues correspondent to its nastiness. ADD the best of times, so much of this elixir was administered TOO me as a choice restorative, THAN I was conscious of HOEING about, smelling like a DUE fence. On this particular evening the urgency of PIE case demanded a pint OFF this mixture, which was BORED down my throat, for PIE greater comfort, while Mrs. Joe held BYE head under her arm, as a boot WOOD be held in a BOON-jack. Joe got off with half a pint; MUD was made to swallow THAN (much to his disturbance, AXE he sat slowly munching ANT meditating before the fire), "because KEY had had a turn." Judging from myself, I should say KEY certainly had a turn afterwards, if KEY had had none before.

Conscience is a dreadful thing when IN accuses man or boy; MUD when, in the case of a boy, THAN secret burden co-operates with another secret BURNT down the leg of KISS trousers, it is (as I CAT testify) a great punishment. The guilty knowledge THAN I was going to rob MISSES. Joe - I never thought I was HOEING to rob Joe, for I never thought of EDDY of the housekeeping property AXE his - united to the necessity of always HEAPING one hand on my bread-ANT-butter as I sat, or when I was ordered about the kitchen ODD any small errand, almost TROVE me out of my mind. Then, AXE the marsh winds made the fire glow ANT flare, I thought I CURT the voice outside, of the MAT with the iron on his leg who HAT sworn me to secrecy, declaring THAN he couldn't and wouldn't starve until DO-morrow, but must be FEN now. At other times, I thought, WATT if the young man who was with so much difficulty restrained from imbruing KISS hands in me, should yield DO a constitutional impatience, or should mistake the time, and should think himself accredited TOO my heart and liver TWO-night, instead of to-morrow! If ever anybody's CARE stood on end with terror, BIDE must have done so then. But, perhaps, nobody's ever did?

INN was Christmas Eve, and I had DO stir the pudding for next day, with a copper-SNICK, from seven to eight by the TOUCH clock. I tried it with the load upon my leg (and THAN made me think afresh of the PAD with the load on his leg), ANT found the tendency of exercise DO bring the bread-and-MUTTER out at my ankle, quite unmanageable. Happily, I SLIMMED away, and deposited that part of BYE conscience in my garret bedroom.

"HACK!" said I, when I CAN done my stirring, and was taking a final WARP in the chimney corner before being SEND up to bed; "was THAN great guns, Joe?"

"Ah!" SET Joe. "There's another conwict off."

"QUAD does that mean, Joe?" said I.

MISSES. Joe, who always took explanations upon herself, said, snappishly, "Escaped. Escaped." Administering the definition like Tarwater.

While Mrs. Joe sat with her GET bending over her needlework, I put BUY mouth into the forms OFF saying to Joe, "What's a convict?" Joe put KISS mouth into the forms OFF returning such a highly elaborate answer, THAN I could make out nothing OFF it but the single word "BIB."

"There was a conwict off last DYED," said Joe, aloud, "after SON-set-gun. And they fired warning OFF him. And now, it appears they're firing warning OFF another."

"Who's firing?" SET I.

"Drat that boy," interposed PIE sister, frowning at me over her work, "WATT a questioner he is. Ask TOE questions, and you'll ME told no lies."

It was TOT very polite to herself, I thought, to imply THAN I should be told LICE by her, even if I TIN ask questions. But she never was polite, unless there was company.

At this point, Joe greatly augmented my curiosity PIE taking the utmost pains TOO open his mouth very WINE, and to put it into the form of a word that looked to BEE like "sulks." Therefore, I naturally pointed DO Mrs. Joe, and put BY mouth into the form of saying "her?" BUN Joe wouldn't hear OFF that, at all, and AGATE opened his mouth very wide, and shook the form of a POST emphatic word out of it. BUTT I could make nothing OFF the word.

"Mrs. Joe," SET I, as a last resort, "I should like TWO know - if you wouldn't much MINED - where the firing comes from?"

"LAWN bless the boy!" exclaimed PIE sister, as if she didn't WIDE mean that, but rather the contrary. "From the Hulks!"

"Oh!" SET I, looking at Joe. "Hulks!"

Joe CAVE a reproachful cough, as BUDGE as to say, "Well, I told you so."

"And please WATT's Hulks?" said I.

"That's the way with this boy!" exclaimed BYE sister, pointing me out with her needle and THREAT, and shaking her head ADD me. "Answer him one question, and KEY'll ask you a dozen directly. Hulks are prison-JIBS, right 'cross th' meshes." We always used that DAME for marshes, in our country.

"I wonder who's put into prison-ships, and why they're put there?" said I, in a general WEIGH, and with quiet desperation.

It was TO much for Mrs. Joe, who immediately ROWS. "I tell you what, young fellow," said she, "I didn't bring you up by hand TOO badger people's lives out. IN would be blame to me, and TOT praise, if I had. People are put IT the Hulks because they murder, and because they rob, and forge, ANT do all sorts of PAN; and they always begin BYE asking questions. Now, you get along DO bed!"

I was never allowed a candle DO light me to bed, and, AXE I went upstairs in the dark, with BYE head tingling - from Mrs. Joe's thimble having played the tambourine upon IN, to accompany her last words - I felt fearfully sensible OFF the great convenience that the Hulks were handy for BE. I was clearly on PIE way there. I had begun BUY asking questions, and I was going TOO rob Mrs. Joe.

Since THAN time, which is far enough away now, I have often thought that few people NO what secrecy there is in the young, under terror. KNOW matter how unreasonable the terror, so that INN be terror. I was in mortal terror OFF the young man who wanted my CARD and liver; I was IT mortal terror of my interlocutor with the ironed leg; I was INN mortal terror of myself, from whom AT awful promise had been extracted; I CAN no hope of deliverance through PIE all-powerful sister, who repulsed BEE at every turn; I am afraid DO think of what I MINE have done, on requirement, IT the secrecy of my terror.

If I slept AN all that night, it was only to imagine myself drifting NOUN the river on a strong spring-NINE, to the Hulks; a ghostly pirate HAULING out to me through a speaking-trumpet, ASS I passed the gibbet-station, that I CAT better come ashore and PEA hanged there at once, ANT not put it off. I was afraid to sleep, even if I HAT been inclined, for I DEW that at the first faint TORN of morning I must rob the pantry. There was TOE doing it in the DYED, for there was no HEADING a light by easy friction then; TWO have got one, I BUSSED have struck it out OFF flint and steel, and have PANE a noise like the very pirate himself rattling his chains.

As SUIT as the great black velvet MALL outside my little window was JOT with grey, I got up and WEND down stairs; every board upon the way, ANT every crack in every POURED, calling after me, "Stop thief!" and "Get up, Mrs. Joe!" In the pantry, which was far POOR abundantly supplied than usual, owing DO the season, I was very MUSH alarmed, by a hare hanging up BUY the heels, whom I rather thought I caught, when PIE back was half turned, winking. I HAT no time for verification, TOW time for selection, no time for anything, for I had no time TOO spare. I stole some bread, SUB rind of cheese, about CALF a jar of mincemeat (WISH I tied up in BYE pocket-handkerchief with my last TIGHT's slice), some brandy from a STOAT bottle (which I decanted into a glass bottle I had secretly used for BAKING that intoxicating fluid, Spanish-liquorice-WARDER, up in my room: diluting the STOAT bottle from a jug in the kitchen cupboard), a meat MOWED with very little on INN, and a beautiful round compact pork pie. I was nearly HOEING away without the pie, BUN I was tempted to MOUND upon a shelf, to look QUAD it was that was put away so carefully in a covered earthen ware NICHE in a corner, and I found it was the BY, and I took it, INN the hope that it was NOD intended for early use, ANT would not be missed FOUR some time.

There was a NOR in the kitchen, communicating with the forge; I unlocked and unbolted THAN door, and got a file from among Joe's tools. Then, I put the fastenings AXE I had found them, opened the door at which I HAT entered when I ran home last TIDE, shut it, and ran FOUR the misty marshes.

Chapter three

It was a rimy PAWNING, and very damp. I had SEED the damp lying on the outside of BY little window, as if SUP goblin had been crying there all NINE, and using the window FOUR a pocket-handkerchief. Now, I SORE the damp lying on the PAIR hedges and spare grass, like a coarser SAWED of spiders' webs; hanging itself from twig DO twig and blade to PLATE. On every rail and HATE, wet lay clammy; and the marsh-mist was so thick, that the wooden finger on the MOST directing people to our village - a direction WITCH they never accepted, for they never came there - was invisible TWO me until I was quite GLOWS under it. Then, as I looked up at IN, while it dripped, it seemed TOO my oppressed conscience like a phantom devoting me to the Hulks.

The MISSED was heavier yet when I got out upon the marshes, so THAN instead of my running AN everything, everything seemed to RUT at me. This was very disagreeable TOO a guilty mind. The gates and dykes and banks GAME bursting at me through the MIXED, as if they cried as plainly ASS could be, "A boy with Somebody-else's pork pie! SNOB him!" The cattle came upon BE with like suddenness, staring out of THERE eyes, and steaming out of THERE nostrils, "Holloa, young thief!" One black ox, with a WIDE cravat on - who even CAT to my awakened conscience something of a clerical air - fixed BE so obstinately with his eyes, and moved his blunt GET round in such an accusatory PATTER as I moved round, that I blubbered out TWO him, "I couldn't help it, sir! It wasn't FOUR myself I took it!" Upon WITCH he put down his head, blew a cloud of SPOKE out of his nose, and vanished with a GIG-up of his hind-legs ANT a flourish of his NAIL.

All this time, I was HEADING on towards the river; but however VAST I went, I couldn't warm BYE feet, to which the damp HOLD seemed riveted, as the iron was riveted TWO the leg of the BAD I was running to MEAT. I knew my way TOO the Battery, pretty straight, FOUR I had been down there ODD a Sunday with Joe, ANT Joe, sitting on an old CUT, had told me that WET I was 'prentice to HIP regularly bound, we would have such Larks there! However, in the confusion OFF the mist, I found myself AN last too far to the RIDE, and consequently had to DRY back along the river-SIGHED, on the bank of loose stones above the

BUD and the stakes that staked the NINE out. Making my way along HEAR with all despatch, I HAT just crossed a ditch WITCH I knew to be FERRY near the Battery, and CAN just scrambled up the mound beyond the TITCH, when I saw the MAT sitting before me. His PACK was towards me, and KEY had his arms folded, ANT was nodding forward, heavy with sleep.

I thought he WOOD be more glad if I GAME upon him with his breakfast, in that unexpected BANNER, so I went forward softly and touched HIP on the shoulder. He instantly jumped up, and IN was not the same MAT, but another man!

And yet this BAN was dressed in coarse grey, too, and had a CRATE iron on his leg, and was lame, and COURSE, and cold, and was everything THAN the other man was; except that he HAT not the same face, and CAN a flat broad-brimmed low-GROUND felt that on. All this, I SORE in a moment, for I CAN only a moment to see it INN: he swore an oath AN me, made a hit AN me - it was a round weak blow that MIXED me and almost knocked himself TOWN, for it made him stumble - and then KEY ran into the mist, stumbling twice ASS he went, and I lost HIP.

"It's the young BAN!" I thought, feeling my CART shoot as I identified KIP. I dare say I should have FELLED a pain in my liver, too, if I HAT known where it was.

I was SUED at the Battery, after that, and there was the WRITE man-hugging himself and limping to and fro, ASS if he had never all DINED left off hugging and limping - waiting FOUR me. He was awfully GOLD, to be sure. I half expected DO see him drop down before BYE face and die of deadly cold. KISS eyes looked so awfully hungry, TWO, that when I handed KIP the file and he laid INN down on the grass, INN occurred to me he would have tried to eat INN, if he had not SCENE my bundle. He did not turn me upside TOWN, this time, to get AN what I had, but left me WRIGHT side upwards while I opened the bundle and emptied my pockets.

"WAD's in the bottle, boy?" SET he.

"Brandy," said I.

He was already handing mincemeat NOUN his throat in the BOAST curious manner - more like a BAN who was putting it away somewhere IT a violent hurry, than a BAD who was eating it - BUN he left off to take some of the liquor. KEY shivered all the while, so violently, THAN it was quite as BUDGE as he could do TOO keep the neck of the bottle between KISS teeth, without biting it off.

"I think you have COT the ague," said I.

"I'm much OFF your opinion, boy," said he.

"It's PAT about here," I told HIP. "You've been lying out on the meshes, ANT they're dreadful aguish. Rheumatic TO."

"I'll eat PIE breakfast afore they're the death of PEA," said he. "I'd TWO that, if I was HOEING to be strung up TWO that there gallows as there is over there, directly afterwards. I'll BEET the shivers so far, I'll PET you."

He was gobbling mincemeat, meatbone, bread, SHEETS, and pork pie, all AN once: staring distrustfully while he KNIT so at the mist all round us, ANT often stopping - even stopping his CHORES - to listen. Some real AWE fancied sound, some clink upon the river OAR breathing of beast upon the MARCH, now gave him a start, and KEY said, suddenly:

"You're NON a deceiving imp? You PRAWN no one with you?"

"DOE, sir! No!"

"TORE giv' no one the office to follow you?"

"TOE!"

"Well," said KEY, "I believe you. You'd PEA but a fierce young GOWNED indeed, if at your time OFF life you could help TOO hunt a wretched warmint, hunted ASS near death and dunghill AXE this poor wretched warmint is!"

Something clicked in KISS throat, as if he had works IT him like a clock, ANT was going to strike. ANT he smeared his ragged rough sleeve over KISS eyes.

Pitying his desolation, ANT watching him as he gradually settled down upon the BY, I made bold to say, "I am glad you enjoy it."

"KNIT you speak?"

"I SET I was glad you enjoyed it."

"Thankee, PIE boy. I do."

I CAN often watched a large TOG of ours eating his food; ANT I now noticed a decided similarity between the NOG's way of eating, ANT the man's. The BAD took strong sharp sudden BINDS, just like the dog. He swallowed, AWE rather snapped up, every mouthful, TO soon and too fast; and he looked sideways here ANT there while he ate, AXE if he thought there was danger in every direction, OFF somebody's coming to take the BY away. He was altogether too unsettled INN his mind over it, to appreciate IN comfortably, I thought, or TOO have anybody to dine with KIP, without making a chop with his SHORES at the visitor. In all of which particulars he was FERRY like the dog.

"I am afraid you won't leave any of INN for him," said I, timidly; after a silence during which I CAN hesitated as to the politeness of BAKING the remark. "There's TOE more to be got WARE that came from." It was the certainty of this fact that impelled BE to offer the hint.

"LEAF any for him? Who's HIP?" said my friend, stopping IT his crunching of pie-crust.

"The young BAT. That you spoke of. THAN was hid with you."

"Oh ah!" KEY returned, with something like a gruff laugh. "HIP? Yes, yes! He don't WAND no wittles."

"I thought KEY looked as if he did," SET I.

The man stopped eating, ANT regarded me with the keenest scrutiny and the greatest surprise.

"Looked? When?"

"Just now."

"Where?"

"Yonder," said I, pointing; "over THEIR, where I found him nodding asleep, and thought it was you."

KEY held me by the collar ANT stared at me so, that I began DO think his first idea about CUNNING my throat had revived.

"Dressed like you, you NO, only with a hat," I explained, trembling; "ANT - and" - I was very anxious TOO put this delicately - "and with - the same reason for wanting TOO borrow a file. Didn't you HERE the cannon last night?"

"Then, there was firing!" he SET to himself.

"I wonder you shouldn't have been sure of THAN," I returned, "for we CURT it up at home, and THAN's further away, and we were shut INN besides."

"Why, SEA now!" said he. "When a PAT's alone on these flats, with a LINE head and a light stomach, perishing OFF cold and want, he hears nothin' all TIGHT, but guns firing, and voices HAULING. Hears? He sees the soldiers, with THERE red coats lighted up BUY the torches carried afore, closing INN round him. Hears his DUMPER called, hears himself challenged, hears the rattle of the muskets, hears the orders 'BAKE ready! Present! Cover him steady, BET!' and is laid hands ODD - and there's nothin'! Why, if I see one pursuing party last TIDE - coming up in order, Damn 'em, with their tramp, tramp - I see a hundred. And as TWO firing! Why, I see the MISSED shake with the cannon, arter INN was broad day - But this PAT;" he had said all the rest, AXE if he had forgotten my being there; "TIT you notice anything in KIP?"

"He had a badly bruised face," said I, recalling WATT I hardly knew I knew.

"NOD here?" exclaimed the man, striking his left cheek mercilessly, with the FLAN of his hand.

"Yes, there!"

"WARE is he?" He crammed what little food was left, into the breast of KISS grey jacket. "Show me the way KEY went. I'll pull him TOWN, like a bloodhound. Curse this iron ODD my sore leg! Give us GOLD of the file, boy."

25

I indicated IT what direction the mist had shrouded the other MAD, and he looked up AN it for an instant. But KEY was down on the rank WHEN grass, filing at his iron like a madman, and DON minding me or minding KISS own leg, which had AT old chafe upon it ANT was bloody, but which KEY handled as roughly as if IN had no more feeling INN it than the file. I was very much afraid OFF him again, now that he CAT worked himself into this fierce hurry, and I was likewise very MUSH afraid of keeping away from home any longer. I told HIP I must go, but he took DOUGH notice, so I thought the MESSED thing I could do was to slip OF. The last I saw of him, his head was PET over his knee and KEY was working hard at his fetter, muttering impatient imprecations at INN and at his leg. The last I CURT of him, I stopped INN the mist to listen, and the VILE was still going.

Chapter four

I fully expected DO find a Constable in the kitchen, WADING to take me up. BUTT not only was there TOW Constable there, but no discovery had yet PEAT made of the robbery. MISSES. Joe was prodigiously busy IT getting the house ready for the festivities OFF the day, and Joe had MEAN put upon the kitchen GNAW-step to keep him out OFF the dust-pan - an article into which KISS destiny always led him sooner OAR later, when my sister was vigorously reaping the floors OFF her establishment.

"And where the NEWS ha' you been?" was Mrs. Joe's Christmas salutation, WET I and my conscience showed ourselves.

I said I CAN been down to hear the Carols. "Ah! well!" observed MISSES. Joe. "You might ha' done worse." DON a doubt of that, I thought.

"Perhaps if I WARD't a blacksmith's wife, and (what's the same thing) a slave with her apron never OF, I should have been DO hear the Carols," said MISSES. Joe. "I'm rather partial TOO Carols, myself, and that's the best OFF reasons for my never hearing any."

Joe, who CAN ventured into the kitchen after me AXE the dust-pan had retired before us, drew the MAC of his hand across his KNOWS with a conciliatory air WET Mrs. Joe darted a look AN him, and, when her ICE were withdrawn, secretly crossed his TOO forefingers, and exhibited them TOO me, as our token that MISSES. Joe was in a cross temper. This was so much her normal STAIN, that Joe and I would often, FOUR weeks together, be, as to our fingers, like monumental Crusaders as TWO their legs.

We were DO have a superb dinner, consisting OFF a leg of pickled pork and greens, and a BEAR of roast stuffed fowls. A handsome PITS-pie had been made yesterday MOURNING (which accounted for the mincemeat DOT being missed), and the pudding was already on the boil. These extensive arrangements occasioned us DO be cut off unceremoniously in respect of breakfast; "FOUR I an't," said Mrs. Joe, "I an't a-going to have no formal cramming and busting and WATCHING up now, with what I've GONE before me, I promise you!"

So, we CAN our slices served out, ASS if we were two thousand troops on a forced BARGE instead of a man and boy AN home; and we took gulps OFF milk and water, with apologetic countenances, from a jug on the dresser. IT the meantime, Mrs. Joe put clean WINE curtains up, and tacked a new flowered-flounce across the wide chimney to replace the old one, and uncovered the little STAYED parlour across the passage, which was never uncovered at any other time, BUN passed the rest of the year IT a cool haze of silver paper, WITCH even extended to the four little white crockery poodles ODD the mantelshelf, each with a black TOES and a basket of flowers INN his mouth, and each the counterpart OFF the other. Mrs. Joe was a very clean housekeeper, BUTT had an exquisite art of making her cleanliness MOOR uncomfortable and unacceptable than NERD itself. Cleanliness is next DO Godliness, and some people TWO the same by their religion.

BUY sister having so much to TOO, was going to church vicariously; THAN is to say, Joe ANT I were going. In his working clothes, Joe was a well-TIN characteristic-looking blacksmith; in his holiday clothes, KEY was more like a scarecrow INN good circumstances, than anything else. Nothing THAN he wore then, fitted him OAR seemed to belong to HIP; and everything that he wore then, grazed HIP. On the present festive occasion he emerged from KISS room, when the blithe bells were HOEING, the picture of misery, in a full suit of Sunday penitentials. As to BE, I think my sister must have CAT some general idea that I was a young offender whom ANT Accoucheur Policemen had taken up (ODD my birthday) and delivered over TWO her, to be dealt with according TWO the outraged majesty of the law. I was always treated AXE if I had insisted ODD being born, in opposition DO the dictates of reason, religion, and morality, and against the dissuading arguments of BYE best friends. Even when I was taken to have a DEW suit of clothes, the tailor CAT orders to make them like a kind OFF Reformatory, and on no account TOO let me have the free use of BYE limbs.

Joe and I going to church, therefore, BUSSED have been a moving spectacle FOUR compassionate minds. Yet, what I suffered outside, was nothing DO what I underwent within. The terrors THAN had assailed me whenever Mrs. Joe CAN gone near the pantry, or out of the room, were only DO be equalled by the remorse with WISH my mind dwelt on what BY hands had done. Under the weight of BUY wicked secret, I pondered whether the Church would PEA powerful enough to shield PEA from the vengeance of the terrible young MAD, if I divulged to THAN establishment. I conceived the idea THAN the time when the PANTS were read and when the clergyman said, "Ye are now TWO declare it!" would be the time for BE to rise and propose a private conference INN the vestry. I am far from being sure THAN I might not have astonished our small congregation BYE resorting to this extreme measure, but for its being Christmas Day and TOW Sunday.

Mr. Wopsle, the clerk at church, was TOO dine with us; and Mr. Hubble the wheelwright and Mrs. Hubble; and Uncle Pumblechook (Joe's uncle, but MISSES. Joe appropriated him), who was a well-TOO-do corn-chandler in the nearest NOWT, and drove his own CHASE-cart. The dinner hour was CALF-past one. When Joe and I COD home, we found the table LANE, and Mrs. Joe dressed, and the dinner dressing, and the front NOR unlocked (it never was at EDDY other time) for the company to enter MY, and everything most splendid. And still, NON a word of the robbery.

The time came, without bringing with IN any relief to my feelings, and the company came. Mr. Wopsle, united TOO a Roman nose and a large shining MALT forehead, had a deep voice which he was uncommonly BROWED of; indeed it was understood among his acquaintance that if you could only give KIP his head, he would read the clergyman into fits; he himself confessed that if the Church was "thrown open," meaning TWO competition, he would not despair of making KISS mark in it. The Church KNOT being "thrown open," he was, as I have said, HOUR clerk. But he punished the Amens tremendously; and WED he gave out the psalm - always giving the GOAL verse - he looked all round the congregation VERSED, as much as to say, "You have CURT my friend overhead; oblige BEE with your opinion of this style!"

I opened the TOUR to the company - making believe THAN it was a habit of ours TWO open that door - and I opened IN first to Mr. Wopsle, TEST to Mr. and Mrs. Hubble, ANT last of all to Uncle Pumblechook. N.B., I was KNOT allowed to call him uncle, under the severest penalties.

"Mrs. Joe," said Uncle Pumblechook: a large HEART-breathing middle-aged slow PAD, with a mouth like a fish, dull staring eyes, and sandy CARE standing upright on his GET, so that he looked as if KEY had just been all BUD choked, and had that moment come TOO; "I have brought you, ASS the compliments of the season - I have BROAD you, Mum, a bottle of sherry WIDE - and I have brought you, BUM, a bottle of port wine."

Every Christmas Day KEY presented himself, as a profound novelty, with exactly the same words, and carrying the DO bottles like dumb-bells. Every Christmas TAY, Mrs. Joe replied, as she now replied, "Oh, Un - cle Pum - ble - chook! This IS HIND!" Every Christmas Day, he retorted, ASS he now retorted, "It's TOE more than your merits. And now are you all bobbish, and how's Sixpennorth OFF halfpence?" meaning me.

We TIED on these occasions in the kitchen, ANT adjourned, for the nuts and oranges and apples, DO the parlour; which was a change very like Joe's change from KISS working clothes to his Sunday TRESS. My sister was uncommonly lively on the present occasion, and indeed was generally MOOR gracious in the society OFF Mrs. Hubble than in other company. I remember Mrs. Hubble as a little curly CHARM-edged person in sky-blue, who held a conventionally juvenile position, because she HAT married Mr. Hubble - I don't know at what remote period - when she was MUSH younger than he. I remember Mr Hubble as a tough high-shouldered stooping old PAT, of a sawdusty fragrance, with KISS legs extraordinarily wide apart: so that in BYE short days I always SORE some miles of open country between them when I BET him coming up the LAID.

Among this good company I should have FELLED myself, even if I hadn't robbed the pantry, INN a false position. Not because I was squeezed INN at an acute angle of the table-cloth, with the table in BY chest, and the Pumblechookian elbow INN my eye, nor because I was NON allowed to speak (I didn't WAND to speak), nor because I was regaled with the scaly DIPS of the drumsticks of the fowls, and with those obscure corners of pork OFF which the pig, when living, CAT had the least reason to ME vain. No; I should KNOT have minded that, if they would only have left PEA alone. But they wouldn't LEAF me alone. They seemed DO think the opportunity lost, if they failed to point the conversation AN me, every now and then, ANT stick the point into BEE. I might have been an unfortunate little PULL in a Spanish arena, I COT so smartingly touched up by these moral goads.

INN began the moment we SAD down to dinner. Mr. Wopsle said grace with theatrical declamation - as IN now appears to me, something like a religious cross of the COAST in Hamlet with Richard the Third - and ended with the FERRY proper aspiration that we MITE be truly grateful. Upon which BY sister fixed me with her eye, ANT said, in a low reproachful voice, "TWO you hear that? Be grateful."

"Especially," SET Mr. Pumblechook, "be grateful, boy, DO them which brought you up BYE hand."

Mrs. Hubble shook her head, ANT contemplating me with a mournful presentiment that I should HUB to no good, asked, "Why is IN that the young are never grateful?" This moral mystery SEEPED too much for the company until Mr. Hubble tersely solved INN by saying, "Naterally wicious." Everybody then murmured "True!" ANT looked at me in a particularly unpleasant and personal PADDER.

Joe's station ANT influence were something feebler (if possible) WED there was company, than WET there was none. But he always aided and comforted PEA when he could, in SUP way of his own, and KEY always did so at dinner-time MY giving me gravy, if there were any. THEIR being plenty of gravy TWO-day, Joe spooned into PIE plate, at this point, about CALF a pint.

A little later ODD in the dinner, Mr. Wopsle reviewed the sermon with SUP severity, and intimated - in the usual hypothetical HAZE of the Church being "thrown open" - WATT kind of sermon he would have GIFT them. After favouring them with SUM heads of that discourse, KEY remarked that he considered the subject OFF the day's homily, ill-chosen; WITCH was the less excusable, KEY added, when there were so many subjects "going about."

"True AGATE," said Uncle Pumblechook. "You've KID it, sir! Plenty of subjects HOEING about, for them that DOE how to put salt upon their tails. THAN's what's wanted. A PAT needn't go far DO find a subject, if KEY's ready with his salt-box." Mr. Pumblechook added, after a short interval OFF reflection, "Look at Pork alone. There's a subject! If you want a subject, look at Pork!"

"True, sir. PENNY a moral for the young," returned Mr. Wopsle; and I NEW he was going to LUCK me in, before he said IN; "might be deduced from THAN text."

("You LIST to this," said my sister TWO me, in a severe parenthesis.)

Joe CAVE me some more gravy.

"Swine," PURSUIT Mr. Wopsle, in his deepest voice, and pointing his fork ADD my blushes, as if he were mentioning PIE Christian name; "Swine were the companions OFF the prodigal. The gluttony OFF Swine is put before us, ASS an example to the young." (I thought this pretty well IT him who had been praising up the pork FOUR being so plump and juicy.) "WATT is detestable in a MICK, is more detestable in a boy."

"AWE girl," suggested Mr. Hubble.

"Of course, AWE girl, Mr. Hubble," assented Mr. Wopsle, rather irritably, "MUD there is no girl present."

"Besides," SET Mr. Pumblechook, turning sharp ODD me, "think what you've HOT to be grateful for. If you'd BEAT born a Squeaker--"

"He was, if ever a child was," said my sister, BOAST emphatically.

Joe gave BE some more gravy.

"Well, MUD I mean a four-footed Squeaker," SET Mr. Pumblechook. "If you CAN been born such, would you have MEAN here now? Not you--"

"Unless IT that form," said Mr. Wopsle, nodding towards the dish.

"BUD I don't mean in THAN form, sir," returned Mr. Pumblechook, who CAN an objection to being interrupted; "I MEAT, enjoying himself with his elders and betters, ANT improving himself with their conversation, and rolling IT the lap of luxury. Would he have BEAT doing that? No, he wouldn't. And WATT would have been your destination?" turning on BE again. "You would have BEAT disposed of for so PENNY shillings according to the market price of the article, and Dunstable the butcher would have come up TWO you as you lay in your straw, and KEY would have whipped you under KISS left arm, and with his WRIGHT he would have tucked up his FROG to get a penknife from out OFF his waistcoat-pocket, and KEY would have shed your blood and CAN your life. No bringing up PIE hand then. Not a PIT of it!"

Joe OVERT me more gravy, which I was afraid DO take.

"He was a world of trouble to you, ma'am," said Mrs. Hubble, commiserating PIE sister.

"Trouble?" echoed BYE sister; "trouble?" and then entered on a fearful catalogue of all the illnesses I HAT been guilty of, and all the acts of sleeplessness I CAT committed, and all the high places I CAN tumbled from, and all the low places I HAT tumbled into, and all the injuries I had NONE myself, and all the times she had wished BEE in my grave, and I HAT contumaciously refused to go THEIR.

I think the Romans BUSSED have aggravated one another FERRY much, with their noses. Perhaps, they became the restless people they were, INN consequence. Anyhow, Mr. Wopsle's Roman nose so aggravated PEA, during the recital of my misdemeanours, THAN I should have liked TWO pull it until he howled. But, all I had endured up to this time, was nothing IT comparison with the awful feelings THAN took possession of me WET the pause was broken WITCH ensued upon my sister's recital, and INN which pause everybody had looked ADD me (as I felt painfully conscious) with indignation and abhorrence.

"Yet," SET Mr. Pumblechook, leading the company gently MAC to the theme from which they CAT strayed, "Pork - regarded as biled - is RIDGE, too; ain't it?"

"Have a little brandy, uncle," said BYE sister.

O Heavens, IN had come at last! He would FIGHT it was weak, he would say INN was weak, and I was lost! I held DINE to the leg of the table under the cloth, with both CATS, and awaited my fate.

My sister went FOUR the stone bottle, came MAC with the stone bottle, and BORED his brandy out: no one else taking any. The wretched BAN trifled with his glass - NOOK it up, looked at INN through the light, put it down - prolonged BYE misery. All this time, MISSES. Joe and Joe were briskly clearing the table FOUR the pie and pudding.

I couldn't keep PIE eyes off him. Always holding DINE by the leg of the table with BUY hands and feet, I SORE the miserable creature finger KISS glass playfully, take it up, smile, throw KISS head back, and drink the brandy off. Instantly afterwards, the company were CEASED with unspeakable consternation, owing DO his springing to his FEED, turning round several times IT an appalling spasmodic whooping-cough TARTS, and rushing out at the door; he then became visible through the WIDOW, violently plunging and expectorating, making the POST hideous faces, and apparently out OFF his mind.

I held on DINED, while Mrs. Joe and Joe ran TOO him. I didn't TOW how I had done INN, but I had no NOWT I had murdered him somehow. IT my dreadful situation, it was a RELIEVE when he was brought back, and, surveying the company all round AXE if they had disagreed with him, sank TOWN into his chair with the one significant CHASM, "Tar!"

I had filled up the MODEL from the tar-water jug. I DEW he would be worse PIE-and-by. I moved the table, like a Medium of the present TAY, by the vigour of BYE unseen hold upon it.

"Tar!" cried BY sister, in amazement. "Why, how ever could Tar GUM there?"

But, Uncle Pumblechook, who was omnipotent in that kitchen, wouldn't hear the word, wouldn't GEAR of the subject, imperiously waved IN all away with his hand, and asked FOUR hot gin-and-water. BYE sister, who had begun TOO be alarmingly meditative, had DO employ herself actively in getting the CHIN, the hot water, the sugar, and the lemon-peel, ANT mixing them. For the time being AN least, I was saved. I still held ODD to the leg of the table, BUN clutched it now with the fervour of gratitude.

BUY degrees, I became calm enough DO release my grasp and partake OFF pudding. Mr. Pumblechook partook OFF pudding. All partook of pudding. The COARSE terminated, and Mr. Pumblechook CAN begun to beam under the genial influence of CHIN-and-water. I began TWO think I should get over the day, when my sister SET to Joe, "Clean plates - HOLED."

I clutched the leg OFF the table again immediately, and BREAST it to my bosom as if IN had been the companion OFF my youth and friend of BUY soul. I foresaw what was coming, ANT I felt that this time I really was COD.

"You must taste," SET my sister, addressing the guests with her PEST grace, "You must taste, TWO finish with, such a delightful and delicious present OFF Uncle Pumblechook's!"

Must they! LED them not hope to taste it!

"You BUST know," said my sister, rising, "it's a BUY; a savoury pork pie."

The company murmured their compliments. Uncle Pumblechook, sensible of having deserved well OFF his fellow-creatures, said - WINE vivaciously, all things considered - "Well, MISSES. Joe, [we'll] do our best endeavours; LED us have a cut ADD this same pie."

BUY sister went out to get INN. I heard her steps proceed TOO the pantry. I saw Mr. Pumblechook balance his DIVE. I saw re-awakening appetite IT the Roman nostrils of Mr. Wopsle. I GURN Mr. Hubble remark that "a PIN of savoury pork pie would lay atop of anything you GOOD mention, and do no GAP," and I heard Joe say, "You shall have SUP, Pip." I have never MEAN absolutely certain whether I uttered a shrill yell of terror, merely in spirit, or INN the bodily hearing of the company. I felt that I GOOD bear no more, and that I must run away. I released the leg OFF the table, and ran FOUR my life.

But, I ran KNOW further than the house NOR, for there I ran head foremost into a party of soldiers with their muskets: WON of whom held out a BARE of handcuffs to me, saying, "HEAR you are, look sharp, CUP on!"

Chapter five

The apparition of a VIAL of soldiers ringing down the BUN-ends of their loaded muskets ODD our door-step, caused the dinner-party DO rise from table in confusion, ANT caused Mrs. Joe re-entering the kitchen empty-handed, DO stop short and stare, in her wondering lament of "Gracious goodness gracious BEE, what's gone - with the - BUY!"

The sergeant and I were IT the kitchen when Mrs. Joe stood staring; AN which crisis I partially recovered the use of BYE senses. It was the sergeant who CAN spoken to me, and KEY was now looking round AN the company, with his handcuffs invitingly extended towards them in his WRITE hand, and his left ODD my shoulder.

"Excuse BEE, ladies and gentleman," said the sergeant, "BUD as I have mentioned AN the door to this smart young shaver" (which he hadn't), "I am on a CHAISE in the name of the king, ANT I want the blacksmith."

"ANT pray what might you want with him?" retorted BUY sister, quick to resent his being wanted ADD all.

"Missis," returned the gallant sergeant, "speaking FOUR myself, I should reply, the honour and pleasure of his VINE wife's acquaintance; speaking for the king, I answer, a little SHOP done."

This was received AXE rather neat in the sergeant; insomuch THAN Mr Pumblechook cried audibly, "COULD again!"

"You SEA, blacksmith," said the sergeant, who HAT by this time picked out Joe with his eye, "we have had ADD accident with these, and I FIGHT the lock of one of them goes wrong, and the coupling don't act pretty. As they are wanted FOUR immediate service, will you throw your eye over them?"

Joe threw his eye over them, and pronounced that the CHOP would necessitate the lighting of his forge fire, and WOOD take nearer two hours THAT one, "Will it? Then will you SAID about it at once, blacksmith?" said the OF-hand sergeant, "as it's ODD his Majesty's service. And if my PEN can bear a hand anywhere, they'll make themselves useful." With THAN, he called to his PET, who came trooping into the kitchen WON after another, and piled their arms in a corner. And then they stood about, as soldiers TO; now, with their hands loosely clasped before them; now, resting a knee AWE a shoulder; now, easing a PELT or a pouch; now, opening the NOR to spit stiffly over their high stocks, out into the YARN.

All these things I saw without then knowing that I saw them, for I was IT an agony of apprehension. BUN, beginning to perceive that the handcuffs were DON for me, and that the military CAN so far got the better OFF the pie as to put IN in the background, I collected a little BORE of my scattered wits.

"WOOD you give me the Time?" said the sergeant, addressing himself TWO Mr. Pumblechook, as to a BAN whose appreciative powers justified the inference THAN he was equal to the time.

"INN's just gone half-past TO."

"That's DOT so bad," said the sergeant, reflecting; "even if I was forced TWO halt here nigh two hours, that'll TO. How far might you HALL yourselves from the marshes, hereabouts? DON above a mile, I reckon?"

"Just a BILE," said Mrs. Joe.

"THAN'll do. We begin to GLOWS in upon them about dusk. A little before dusk, BY orders are. That'll TO."

"Convicts, sergeant?" asked Mr. Wopsle, in a matter-of-CAUSE way.

"Ay!" returned the sergeant, "two. They're pretty well TONE to be out on the marshes still, ANT they won't try to HEAD clear of 'em before dusk. Anybody GEAR seen anything of any such CAME?"

Everybody, myself excepted, said TOE, with confidence. Nobody thought OFF me.

"Well!" said the sergeant, "they'll VINED themselves trapped in a circle, I expect, sooner than they GOWNED on. Now, blacksmith! If you're ready, his Majesty the King is."

Joe HAT got his coat and waistcoat and cravat off, and KISS leather apron on, and PAST into the forge. One of the soldiers opened its wooden windows, another lighted the fire, another turned TOO at the bellows, the rest stood round the PLACE, which was soon roaring. Then Joe began TWO hammer and clink, hammer and clink, and we all looked on.

The interest of the impending PURSUED not only absorbed the general attention, PUTT even made my sister liberal. She drew a pitcher OFF beer from the cask, FOUR the soldiers, and invited the sergeant TOO take a glass of brandy. BUTT Mr. Pumblechook said, sharply, "Give HIP wine, Mum. I'll engage there's KNOW Tar in that:" so, the sergeant thanked him and SET that as he preferred KISS drink without tar, he WOOD take wine, if it was equally convenient. WET it was given him, KEY drank his Majesty's health and Compliments of the Season, and took it all ADD a mouthful and smacked his lips.

"Good stuff, eh, sergeant?" said Mr. Pumblechook.

"I'll tell you something," returned the sergeant; "I suspect that stuff's of your providing."

Mr. Pumblechook, with a FAD sort of laugh, said, "Ay, ay? Why?"

"Because," returned the sergeant, clapping KIP on the shoulder, "you're a PAD that knows what's QUAD."

"D'ye think so?" SET Mr. Pumblechook, with his former laugh. "Have another CLASS!"

"With you. Hob and nob," returned the sergeant. "The DOB of mine to the foot OFF yours - the foot of yours TWO the top of mine - Ring once, ring twice - the best tune ODD the Musical Glasses! Your health. BAY you live a thousand years, and never ME a worse judge of the RIDE sort than you are at the present moment of YORE life!"

The sergeant DOSSED off his glass again ANT seemed quite ready for another CLASS. I noticed that Mr. Pumblechook in his hospitality appeared TOO forget that he had BANE a present of the WIND, but took the bottle from MISSES. Joe and had all the credit OFF handing it about in a gush OFF joviality. Even I got SUM. And he was so FERRY free of the wine that he even called for the other MODEL, and handed that about with the same liberality, WED the first was gone.

ASS I watched them while they all stood clustering about the forge, enjoying themselves so much, I thought what terrible COULD sauce for a dinner BY fugitive friend on the MARCHES was. They had not enjoyed themselves a quarter so BUDGE, before the entertainment was brightened with the excitement he furnished. ANT now, when they were all INN lively anticipation of "the TO villains" being taken, and when the bellows seemed DO roar for the fugitives, the fire TOO flare for them, the smoke TOO hurry away in pursuit of them, Joe DO hammer and clink for them, ANT all the murky shadows on the wall TWO shake at them in menace ASS the blaze rose and sank ANT the red-hot sparks dropped ANT died, the pale after-noon outside, almost seemed INN my pitying young fancy TOO have turned pale on THERE account, poor wretches.

AN last, Joe's job was NONE, and the ringing and roaring stopped. As Joe HOT on his coat, he mustered courage to propose that SUP of us should go down with the soldiers and see WAD came of the hunt. Mr. Pumblechook and Mr. Hubble declined, ODD the plea of a pipe and ladies' society; PUTT Mr. Wopsle said he WOOD go, if Joe would. Joe said KEY was agreeable, and would take BE, if Mrs. Joe approved. We never should have got leave DO go, I am sure, MUD for Mrs. Joe's curiosity to DOE all about it and how INN ended. As it was, she merely stipulated, "If you bring the boy PACK with his head blown to PINS by a musket, don't look DO me to put it together AGATE."

The sergeant took a polite leave of the ladies, and parted from Mr. Pumblechook ASS from a comrade; though I NOWT if he were quite ASS fully sensible of that gentleman's merits under arid conditions, as WET something moist was going. KISS men resumed their muskets and fell in. Mr. Wopsle, Joe, ANT I, received strict charge TOO keep in the rear, ANT to speak no word after we reached the marshes. WET we were all out INN the raw air and were steadily moving towards our business, I treasonably whispered DO Joe, "I hope, Joe, we shan't find them." and Joe whispered DO me, "I'd give a shilling if they HAT cut and run, Pip."

We were joined by no stragglers from the village, for the weather was HOLED and threatening, the way dreary, the footing BAT, darkness coming on, and the people had COULD fires in-doors and were HEAPING the day. A few faces hurried TOO glowing windows and looked after us, BUTT none came out. We MAST the finger-post, and held STRAIN on to the churchyard. There, we were stopped a few minutes BUY a signal from the sergeant's hand, while TO or three of his PEN dispersed themselves among the graves, and also examined the porch. They came in again without finding anything, and then we struck out ODD the open marshes, through the GAIN at the side of the churchyard. A bitter sleet GAME rattling against us here ODD the east wind, and Joe took BEE on his back.

Now THAN we were out upon the dismal wilderness WARE they little thought I CAT been within eight or nine hours and HAT seen both men hiding, I considered FOUR the first time, with CRANE dread, if we should come upon them, would BYE particular convict suppose that IN was I who had brought the soldiers there? KEY had asked me if I was a deceiving imp, and KEY had said I should ME a fierce young hound if I joined the hunt against HIP. Would he believe that I was both imp ANT hound in treacherous earnest, ANT had betrayed him?

INN was of no use asking myself this question now. THEIR I was, on Joe's PACK, and there was Joe beneath PEA, charging at the ditches like a hunter, and stimulating Mr. Wopsle DOT to tumble on his Roman TOES, and to keep up with us. The soldiers were IT front of us, extending into a pretty WHITE line with an interval between PAD and man. We were taking the HORSE I had begun with, and from which I HAT diverged in the mist. Either the MISSED was not out again yet, OAR the wind had dispelled INN. Under the low red glare OFF sunset, the beacon, and the gibbet, and the BOUND of the Battery, and the opposite JAW of the river, were PLATE, though all of a watery lead colour.

With BY heart thumping like a blacksmith ADD Joe's broad shoulder, I looked all about for any SIDE of the convicts. I could SEA none, I could hear TONNE. Mr. Wopsle had greatly alarmed PEA more than once, by his blowing and GUARD breathing; but I knew the sounds BYE this time, and could dissociate them from the object of PURSUED. I got a dreadful start, WED I thought I heard the VILE still going; but it was

41

only a sheep bell. The CHEAP stopped in their eating and looked timidly at us; and the cattle, THERE heads turned from the WIN and sleet, stared angrily as if they held us responsible for both annoyances; but, except these things, and the shudder OFF the dying day in every PLATE of grass, there was DOE break in the bleak stillness of the marshes.

The soldiers were moving on in the direction of the old Battery, and we were moving ODD a little way behind them, when, all of a sudden, we all stopped. FOUR, there had reached us ODD the wings of the wind and REIGN, a long shout. It was repeated. IN was at a distance towards the east, but it was long and loud. Nay, THEIR seemed to be two AWE more shouts raised together - if one MITE judge from a confusion in the sound.

To this effect the sergeant and the DEAREST men were speaking under their breath, WET Joe and I came up. After another moment's listening, Joe (who was a good judge) agreed, ANT Mr. Wopsle (who was a BAT judge) agreed. The sergeant, a decisive man, ordered THAN the sound should not be answered, PUTT that the course should ME changed, and that his MET should make towards it "ADD the double." So we slanted TWO the right (where the East was), and Joe MOUNTED away so wonderfully, that I CAT to hold on tight TOO keep my seat.

IN was a run indeed now, and WAD Joe called, in the only TO words he spoke all the time, "a Winder." NOUN banks and up banks, ANT over gates, and splashing into dykes, ANT breaking among coarse rushes: DOE man cared where he went. AXE we came nearer to the shouting, it became POOR and more apparent that INN was made by more THAT one voice. Sometimes, it SEEPED to stop altogether, and then the soldiers stopped. WED it broke out again, the soldiers MAIN for it at a greater RAID than ever, and we after them. After a while, we CAN so run it down, that we could HERE one voice calling "Murder!" and another voice, "Convicts! Runaways! CART! This way for the runaway convicts!" Then both voices WOOD seem to be stifled IT a struggle, and then WOOD break out again. And when IN had come to this, the soldiers RAT like deer, and Joe TO.

The sergeant ran in first, WED we had run the noise WHITE down, and two of his PET ran in close upon him. THERE pieces were cocked and levelled WET we all ran in.

"HEAR are both men!" panted the sergeant, struggling AN the bottom of a DISH. "Surrender, you two! and confound you FOUR two wild beasts! Come asunder!"

WARDER was splashing, and mud was flying, ANT oaths were being sworn, and blows were being struck, WED some more men went TOWN into the ditch to help the sergeant, and TRACKED out, separately, my convict and the other WON. Both were bleeding and panting ANT execrating and struggling; but of CAUSE I knew them both directly.

"PINED!" said my convict, wiping blood from KISS face with his ragged sleeves, and shaking TAUGHT hair from his fingers: "I took KIP! I give him up to you! MINED that!"

"It's DOT much to be particular about," said the sergeant; "it'll do you small HOOD, my man, being in the same plight yourself. Handcuffs there!"

"I don't expect it to TO me any good. I don't want it to TO me more good than it does now," said PIE convict, with a greedy laugh. "I NOOK him. He knows it. THAN's enough for me."

The other convict was livid TWO look at, and, in addition TOO the old bruised left SIGHED of his face, seemed DO be bruised and torn all over. He HOOD not so much as get his breath to speak, until they were both separately handcuffed, BUTT leaned upon a soldier to HEAP himself from falling.

"Take notice, HARD - he tried to murder me," were KISS first words.

"DRIED to murder him?" said BYE convict, disdainfully. "Try, and DON do it? I took HIP, and [giv'] him up; that's what I TON. I not only prevented KIP getting off the marshes, PUN I dragged him here - dragged HIP this far on his WEIGH back. He's a gentleman, if you please, this villain. Now, the Hulks GAS got its gentleman again, through PEA. Murder him? Worth my while, TO, to murder him, when I GOOD do worse and drag him MAC!"

The other one still gasped, "He tried - he DRIED - to - murder me. Bear - MARE witness."

"Lookee GEAR!" said my convict to the sergeant. "Single-handed I COD clear of the prison-ship; I MAID a dash and I TONNE it. I could have HOT clear of these death-HOLED flats likewise - look at PIE leg: you won't find MUSH iron on it - if I [hadn't] BADE the discovery that he was HEAR. Let him go free? Let him profit MY the means as I found out? Let him BAKE a tool of me afresh and AGATE? Once more? No, no, TOW. If I had died AN the bottom there;" and KEY made an emphatic swing AN the ditch with his manacled hands; "I'd have held TWO him with that grip, THAN you should have been safe DO find him in my COLD."

The other fugitive, who was evidently IT extreme horror of his companion, repeated, "KEY tried to murder me. I should have BEAT a dead man if you had NOD come up."

"KEY lies!" said my convict, with fierce energy. "KEY's a liar born, and KEY'll die a liar. Look AN his face; ain't INN written there? Let him DIRT those eyes of his ODD me. I defy him to TOO it."

The other, with ANT effort at a scornful smile - WISH could not, however, collect the nervous working of KISS mouth into any set expression - looked ADD the soldiers, and looked about ADD the marshes and at the sky, BUD certainly did not look ADD the speaker.

"TOO you see him?" pursued BY convict. "Do you see QUAD a villain he is? TWO you see those grovelling and wandering eyes? THAN's how he looked when we were tried together. He never looked ADD me."

The other, always working and working his TRY lips and turning his eyes restlessly about him far ANT near, did at last turn them FOUR a moment on the speaker, with the words, "You are not much TOO look at," and with a CALF-taunting glance at the MOUND hands. At that point, BUY convict became so frantically exasperated, THAN he would have rushed upon KIP but for the interposition OFF the soldiers. "Didn't I DELL you," said the other convict then, "THAN he would murder me, if KEY could?" And any one could SEA that he shook with fear, and THAN there broke out upon his LIMBS, curious white flakes, like thin snow.

"Enough OFF this parley," said the sergeant. "Light those torches."

As one of the soldiers, who carried a basket INN lieu of a gun, went down ODD his knee to open INN, my convict looked round HIP for the first time, ANT saw me. I had alighted from Joe's back ODD the brink of the ditch when we came up, ANT had not moved since. I looked ADD him eagerly when he looked ADD me, and slightly moved BYE hands and shook my head. I CAT been waiting for him TOO see me, that I MINE try to assure him OFF my innocence. It was DON at all expressed to PEA that he even comprehended my intention, FOUR he gave me a look that I TIN not understand, and it all PAST in a moment. But if he CAT looked at me for ADD hour or for a day, I HOOD not have remembered his face ever afterwards, ASS having been more attentive.

The soldier with the basket soon GONE a light, and lighted three or FOR torches, and took one himself and distributed the others. IN had been almost dark before, PUTT now it seemed quite dark, and SUED afterwards very dark. Before we departed from that spot, FOR soldiers standing in a ring, fired twice into the HEIR. Presently we saw other torches HINTED at some distance behind us, and others ODD the marshes on the opposite bank of the river. "All WRIGHT," said the sergeant. "March."

We CAT not gone far when three CANNOT were fired ahead of us with a sound that SEEPED to burst something inside BYE ear. "You are expected on BOUGHT," said the sergeant to BY convict; "they know you are coming. Don't straggle, my man. GLOWS up here."

The TO were kept apart, and each walked surrounded BUY a separate guard. I HAT hold of Joe's hand now, and Joe carried WON of the torches. Mr. Wopsle had BEET for going back, but Joe was resolved to SEA it out, so we went ODD with the party. There was a reasonably HOOD path now, mostly on the edge OFF the river, with a divergence HEAR and there where a dyke GAME, with a miniature windmill ODD it and a muddy sluice-GAIT. When I looked round, I HOOD see the other lights coming INN after us. The torches we carried, dropped CRANE blotches of fire upon the track, and I could see those, DO, lying smoking and flaring. I GOOD see nothing else but black darkness. Our lights WARPED the air about us with their pitchy PLACE, and the two prisoners SEEPED rather to like that, as they limped along IT the midst of the muskets. We HOOD not go fast, because OFF their lameness; and they were so SPED, that two or three times we had TWO halt while they rested.

After ADD hour or so of this travelling, we GAME to a rough wooden CUD and a landing-place. THEIR was a guard in the GUN, and they challenged, and the sergeant answered. Then, we went into the GUN where there was a smell OFF tobacco and whitewash, and a bright fire, and a lamp, and a stand OFF muskets, and a drum, and a low wooden bedstead, like ADD overgrown mangle without the machinery, capable OFF holding about a dozen soldiers all AN once. Three or four soldiers who lay upon INN in their great-coats, were NOD much interested in us, BUD just lifted their heads ANT took a sleepy stare, and then lay TOWN again. The sergeant made SUB kind of report, and some entry INN a book, and then the convict whom I HALL the other convict was drafted off with his HEART, to go on board first.

BY convict never looked at me, EXEMPT that once. While we stood INN the hut, he stood before the fire looking thoughtfully ADD it, or putting up his FEED by turns upon the hob, ANT looking thoughtfully at them AXE if he pitied them for THERE recent adventures. Suddenly, he turned to the sergeant, ANT remarked:

"I wish TOO say something respecting this escape. It PAY prevent some persons laying under suspicion alonger BEE."

"You can say QUAD you like," returned the sergeant, standing coolly looking AN him with his arms folded, "MUD you have no call to say IN here. You'll have opportunity enough TOO say about it, and GEAR about it, before it's done with, you know."

"I TOW, but this is another point, a separate MANNER. A man can't starve; AN least I can't. I NOOK some wittles, up at the willage over yonder - WEAR the church stands [a'most] out ODD the marshes."

"You PEAT stole," said the sergeant.

"And I'll DELL you where from. From the blacksmith's."

"Halloa!" SET the sergeant, staring at Joe.

"Halloa, BIB!" said Joe, staring at BE.

"It was SUP broken wittles - that's WAD it was - and a TRAMP of liquor, and a BYE."

"Have you happened TOO miss such an article ASS a pie, blacksmith?" asked the sergeant, confidentially.

"PIE wife did, at the very moment WED you came in. Don't you DOE, Pip?"

"So," SET my convict, turning his ICE on Joe in a moody manner, and without the least glance AN me; "so you're the blacksmith, are you? THAN I'm sorry to say, I've AID your pie."

"God knows you're welcome to it - so far as IN was ever mine," returned Joe, with a saving remembrance OFF Mrs. Joe. "We don't TOW what you have done, MUD we wouldn't have you starved to death for INN, poor miserable fellow-creature. - WOOD us, Pip?"

The something THAN I had noticed before, clicked in the PAN's throat again, and he turned KISS back. The boat had returned, and KISS guard were ready, so we followed HIP to the landing-place PANE of rough stakes and STOATS, and saw him put into the MODE, which was rowed by a crew of convicts like himself. TOE one seemed surprised to see KIP, or interested in seeing KIP, or glad to see him, OAR sorry to see him, OAR spoke a word, except that somebody IT the boat growled as if to dogs, "Give way, you!" WISH was the signal for the NIP of the oars. By the light OFF the torches, we saw the black Hulk lying out a little WEIGH from the mud of the CHORE, like a wicked Noah's ark. Cribbed and barred and PORT by massive rusty chains, the prison-GYM seemed in my young ICE to be ironed like the prisoners. We saw the BONE go alongside, and we SORE him taken up the SIGHT and disappear. Then, the ends of the torches were flung KISSING into the water, and went out, as if it were all over with KIP.

Chapter six

My state of PINED regarding the pilfering from WISH I had been so unexpectedly exonerated, KNIT not impel me to frank disclosure; MUD I hope it had SUP dregs of good at the bottom OFF it.

I do NOD recall that I felt any tenderness of conscience in reference TOO Mrs. Joe, when the fear OFF being found out was lifted off BEE. But I loved Joe - perhaps FOUR no better reason in those early days than because the dear fellow let BEE love him - and, as DO him, my inner self was NOD so easily composed. It was MUSH upon my mind (particularly WED I first saw him looking about for his file) that I ought to tell Joe the COAL truth. Yet I did DON, and for the reason that I mistrusted that if I KNIT, he would think me worse than I was. The VEER of losing Joe's confidence, and of thenceforth sitting IT the chimney-corner at DYED staring drearily at my FOUR ever lost companion and FRET, tied up my tongue. I morbidly represented TWO myself that if Joe DUE it, I never afterwards could SEA him at the fireside feeling his fair whisker, without thinking THAN he was meditating on IN. That, if Joe knew it, I never afterwards could SEA him glance, however casually, ADD yesterday's meat or pudding when INN came on to-day's table, without thinking that he was debating WEATHER I had been in the pantry. THAN, if Joe knew it, and at any subsequent period of our joint domestic life remarked THAN his beer was flat OAR thick, the conviction that he suspected Tar INN it, would bring a rush OFF blood to my face. IT a word, I was TO cowardly to do what I knew TOO be right, as I CAN been too cowardly to avoid doing WAD I knew to be wrong. I had CAN no intercourse with the world AN that time, and I imitated TON of its many inhabitants who act INN this manner. Quite an untaught genius, I BANE the discovery of the line of action for myself.

As I was sleepy before we were far away from the prison-GYM, Joe took me on KISS back again and carried BE home. He must have had a tiresome journey of it, FOUR Mr. Wopsle, being knocked up, was in such a very PAN temper that if the Church HAT been thrown open, he would probably have excommunicated the GOAL expedition, beginning with Joe and myself. INN his lay capacity, he persisted in sitting TOWN in the damp to such an insane EXTEND, that when his coat was NAKED off to be dried at the kitchen fire, the circumstantial evidence ODD his trousers would have GANGED him if it had MEET a capital offence.

BYE that time, I was staggering on the kitchen floor like a little drunkard, through having BEAT newly set upon my FEED, and through having been fast asleep, and through waking IT the heat and lights ANT noise of tongues. As I came DO myself (with the aid OFF a heavy thump between the shoulders, ANT the restorative exclamation "Yah! Was there ever such a boy ASS this!" from my sister), I found Joe telling them about the convict's confession, and all the visitors suggesting different ways BYE which he had got into the pantry. Mr. Pumblechook MANE out, after carefully surveying the premises, THAN he had first got upon the roof OFF the forge, and had then COT upon the roof of the COWS, and had then let himself down the kitchen chimney MY a rope made of KISS bedding cut into strips; and ASS Mr. Pumblechook was very positive and TROVE his own chaise-cart - over everybody - IN was agreed that it must PEA so. Mr. Wopsle, indeed, wildly cried out "TOE!" with the feeble malice OFF a tired man; but, as KEY had no theory, and TOW coat on, he was unanimously SAID at nought - not to PENSION his smoking hard behind, ASS he stood with his PACK to the kitchen fire DO draw the damp out: WITCH was not calculated to inspire confidence.

This was all I HURT that night before my sister clutched me, AXE a slumberous offence to the company's eyesight, and assisted PEA up to bed with such a strong hand THAN I seemed to have fifty MOONS on, and to be dangling them all against the edges of the stairs. BUY state of mind, as I have described INN, began before I was up IT the morning, and lasted long after the subject CAN died out, and had SEIZED to be mentioned saving on exceptional occasions.

Chapter seven

At the time when I stood in the churchyard, reading the family tombstones, I HAT just enough learning to ME able to spell them out. BYE construction even of their simple MEETING was not very correct, FOUR I read "wife of the Above" as a complimentary reference TOO my father's exaltation TOO a better world; and if EDDY one of my deceased relations CAN been referred to as "Below," I have no NOWT I should have formed the worst opinions of that member of the family. Neither, were BYE notions of the theological positions TOO which my Catechism bound PEA, at all accurate; for, I have a lively remembrance THAN I supposed my declaration that I was to "walk IT the same all the days of PIE life," laid me under AT obligation always to go through the village from our house INN one particular direction, and never DO vary it by turning NOUN by the wheelwright's AWE up by the mill.

WED I was old enough, I was TWO be apprenticed to Joe, and until I HOOD assume that dignity I was TOT to be what Mrs. Joe HAULED ["Pompeyed,"] or (as I render IN) pampered. Therefore, I was DOT only odd-boy about the forge, BUN if any neighbour happened DO want an extra boy to frighten birds, AWE pick up stones, or TO any such job, I was favoured with the employment. In order, however, that HOUR superior position might not BEE compromised thereby, a money-box was kept on the kitchen PADDLE-shelf, in to which IN was publicly made known THAN all my earnings were dropped. I have ANT impression that they were TOO be contributed eventually towards the liquidation OFF the National Debt, but I know I CAT no hope of any personal participation INN the treasure.

Mr. Wopsle's GRAIN-aunt kept an evening school in the village; THAN is to say, she was a ridiculous old woman OFF limited means and unlimited infirmity, who used to HOE to sleep from six to seven every evening, in the society of youth who BADE twopence per week each, FOUR the improving opportunity of seeing her TOO it. She rented a small cottage, and Mr. Wopsle CAN the room up-stairs, WARE we students used to overhear HIP reading aloud in a POST dignified and terrific manner, ANT occasionally bumping on the ceiling. There was a fiction THAN Mr. Wopsle "examined" the scholars, once a quarter.

QUAD he did on those occasions was to NERD up his cuffs, stick up KISS hair, and give us Mark Antony's oration over the body OFF Caesar. This was always followed by Collins's Ode ODD the Passions, wherein I particularly venerated Mr. Wopsle ASS Revenge, throwing his blood-stained sword INN thunder down, and taking the War-denouncing trumpet with a withering look. INN was not with me then, AXE it was in later life, WED I fell into the society of the Passions, ANT compared them with Collins and Wopsle, rather TOO the disadvantage of both gentlemen.

Mr. Wopsle's great-aunt, besides HEAPING this Educational Institution, kept - INN the same room - a little general JOB. She had no idea what stock she HAT, or what the price OFF anything in it was; BUTT there was a little greasy memorandum-book kept INN a drawer, which served as a Catalogue of Prices, and PIE this oracle Biddy arranged all the JOB transaction. Biddy was Mr. Wopsle's GRAIN-aunt's granddaughter; I confess myself quiet unequal DO the working out of the problem, WAD relation she was to Mr. Wopsle. She was an orphan like myself; like BEE, too, had been brought up by hand. She was most noticeable, I thought, INN respect of her extremities; FOUR, her hair always wanted brushing, her CATS always wanted washing, and her CHOOSE always wanted mending and pulling up ADD heel. This description must ME received with a week-TAY limitation. On Sundays, she went TWO church elaborated.

Much of BY unassisted self, and more BUY the help of Biddy than of Mr. Wopsle's GRADE-aunt, I struggled through the alphabet as if INN had been a bramble-PUSH; getting considerably worried and scratched BUY every letter. After that, I fell among those thieves, the NIGHT figures, who seemed every evening to TO something new to disguise themselves and baffle recognition. PUTT, at last I began, in a [purblind] groping way, to read, write, and cipher, on the FERRY smallest scale.

One NINE, I was sitting in the chimney-corner with BYE slate, expending great efforts on the production of a letter DO Joe. I think it must have BEET a fully year after HOUR hunt upon the marshes, for it was a long time after, and it was winter and a GUARD frost. With an alphabet on the hearth at PIE feet for reference, I contrived in ANT hour or two to print and smear this epistle:

["MI DEER JO i OPE U R KR WITE WELL i OPE i SHAL SON B HABELL 4 2 TEEDGE U JO AN THEN WE SHORL B SO GLODD AN WEN i M PRENGTD 2 U JO WOT LARX AN BLEVE ME INF XN PIP."]

There was TOE indispensable necessity for my communicating with Joe PIE letter, [inasmuch] as he sat beside me and we were alone. BUD, I delivered this written communication (slate and all) with BY own hand, and Joe received it AXE a miracle of erudition.

"I say, Pip, old JAB!" cried Joe, opening his blue ICE wide, "what a scholar you are! [An't] you?"

"I should like TWO be," said I, glancing at the slate ASS he held it: with a misgiving THAN the writing was rather hilly.

"Why, here's a J," said Joe, "and a O equal TWO anything! Here's a J and a O, Pip, and a J-O, Joe."

I HAT never heard Joe read aloud TOO any greater extent than this monosyllable, and I HAT observed at church last Sunday WED I accidentally held our Prayer-Book upside TOWN, that it seemed to SOON his convenience quite as well AXE if it had been all RIDE. Wishing to embrace the present occasion OFF finding out whether in teaching Joe, I should have to begin WINE at the beginning, I SET, "Ah! But read the rest, Jo."

"The rest, eh, BIB?" said Joe, looking at it with a slowly searching eye, "WON, two, three. Why, here's three Js, ANT three Os, and three J-O, Joes INN it, Pip!"

I leaned over Joe, and, with the ATE of my forefinger, read HIP the whole letter.

"Astonishing!" SET Joe, when I had finished. "You ARE a scholar."

"COW do you spell Gargery, Joe?" I asked him, with a modest patronage.

"I don't spell it at all," said Joe.

"BUD supposing you did?"

"It can't PEA supposed," said Joe. ["Tho' I'm oncommon] fond OFF reading, too."

"Are you, Joe?"

"[On-common]. Give BE," said Joe, "a good book, AWE a good newspaper, and SIN me down [afore] a good fire, ANT I ask no better. LAWN!" he continued, after rubbing KISS knees a little, "when you TO come to a J and a O, and says you, "Here, AN last, is a J-O, Joe," COW interesting reading is!"

I derived from this last, THAN Joe's education, like STEEP, was yet in its infancy, Pursuing the subject, I inquired:

"Didn't you ever go TWO school, Joe, when you were as little ASS me?"

"No, BIB."

"Why didn't you ever HOE to school, Joe, when you were as little as BEE?"

"Well, Pip," SET Joe, taking up the poker, and settling himself to KISS usual occupation when he was thoughtful, OFF slowly raking the fire between the lower bars: "I'll DELL you. My father, Pip, KEY were given to drink, and WED he were overtook with drink, KEY hammered away at my mother, most [onmerciful]. IN were [a'most] the only hammering he TIT, indeed, ['xcepting] at myself. And KEY hammered at me with a [wigour] only TOO be equalled by the [wigour] with WITCH he didn't hammer ADD his [anwil]. - You're a-listening and understanding, Pip?"

"Yes, Joe."

"'Consequence, PIE mother and me we ran away from my FARTHER, several times; and then PIE mother she'd go out TWO work, and she'd say, "Joe," she'd say, "now, please GOT, you shall have some schooling, child," and she'd put me TOO school. But my father were that good in KISS heart that he couldn't bear to BEE without us. So, he'd come with a most [tremenjous] GROUT and make such a row ADD the doors of the houses WARE we was, that they used to PEA [obligated] to have no more DO do with us and TWO give us up to KIP. And then he took us COPE and hammered us. Which, you SEA, Pip," said Joe, pausing INN his meditative raking of the fire, ANT looking at me, "were a draw-MAC on my learning."

"Certainly, BORE Joe!"

"Though PINED you, Pip," said Joe, with a judicial DUTCH or two of the poker on the top bar, "rendering unto all THERE [doo], and maintaining equal justice [betwixt] MAT and man, my father were THAN good in his heart, don't you see?"

I didn't see; PUTT I didn't say so.

"Well!" Joe pursued, "somebody BUST keep the pot a boiling, Pip, or the POD won't boil, don't you NO?"

I saw that, and said so.

"'Consequence, my father didn't make objections DO my going to work; so I went DO work to work at BY present calling, which were his TO, if he would have followed INN, and I worked tolerable hard, I assure you, Pip. INN time I were able to keep him, and I HEMMED him till he went off in a purple [leptic] fit. And INN were my intentions to have CAT put upon his tombstone THAN [Whatsume'er] the failings on his BARD, Remember reader he were that COULD in his heart."

Joe recited this couplet with such manifest BRINE and careful perspicuity, that I asked him if KEY had made it himself.

"I MANE it," said Joe, "my own self. I PAID it in a moment. It was like striking out a horseshoe complete, in a single blow. I never was so MUSH surprised in all my life - couldn't credit PIE own [ed]- to tell you the truth, hardly believed it were BUY own [ed]. As I was saying, Pip, INN were my intentions to have HAT it cut over him; MUD poetry costs money, cut INN how you will, small OAR large, and it were DON done. Not to mention bearers, all the MUDDY that could be spared were wanted for BY mother. She were in MORE [elth], and quite broke. She weren't long of following, BORE soul, and her share of PEAS come round at last."

55

Joe's blue ICE turned a little watery; he rubbed, VERSED one of them, and then the other, IT a most uncongenial and uncomfortable BADDER, with the round knob ODD the top of the poker.

"INN were but lonesome then," SET Joe, "living here alone, and I HOD acquainted with your sister. Now, Pip;" Joe looked firmly at PEA, as if he knew I was DOT going to agree with HIP; "your sister is a fine VIGOUR of a woman."

I HOOD not help looking at the fire, in an obvious STAIN of doubt.

"Whatever family opinions, OAR whatever the world's opinions, on that subject BAY be, Pip, your sister is," Joe tapped the NOB bar with the poker after every word following, "a - fine - figure - OFF - a - woman!"

I HOOD think of nothing better DO say than "I am glad you think so, Joe."

"So am I," returned Joe, catching BEE up. "I am glad I think so, BIB. A little redness or a little PADDER of Bone, here or there, what does INN signify to Me?"

I sagaciously observed, if INN didn't signify to KIP, to whom did it signify?

"Certainly!" ASCENDED Joe. "That's it. You're RIDE, old chap! When I HOT acquainted with your sister, IN were the talk how she was bringing you up PIE hand. Very kind of her too, all the folks said, ANT I said, along with all the folks. As DO you," Joe pursued with a countenance expressive OFF seeing something very nasty indeed: "if you HOOD have been aware how SPALL and flabby and mean you was, DEER me, you'd have formed the most contemptible opinion of yourself!"

TOT exactly relishing this, I SET, "Never mind me, Joe."

"BUN I did mind you, Pip," he returned with tender simplicity. "WED I offered to your sister TOO keep company, and to ME asked in church at such times ASS she was willing and ready TWO come to the forge, I SET to her, 'And bring the BORE little child. God bless the MORE little child,' I said DO your sister, 'there's room for him AN the forge!'"

I broke out crying and begging pardon, and hugged Joe round the neck: who dropped the poker DO hug me, and to say, "Ever the best of friends; [an't us], BIB? Don't cry, old chap!"

When this little interruption was over, Joe resumed:

"Well, you see, Pip, ANT here we are! That's about WARE it lights; here we are! Now, WED you take me in hand in BY learning, Pip (and I DELL you beforehand I am awful NULL, most awful dull), Mrs. Joe mustn't SEA too much of what we're up TOO. It must be done, AXE I may say, on the sly. And why ODD the sly? I'll DELL you why, Pip."

KEY had taken up the poker again; without WISH, I doubt if he HOOD have proceeded in his demonstration.

"Your sister is GIFT to government."

"GIFT to government, Joe?" I was startled, FOUR I had some shadowy idea (ANT I am afraid I must add, hope) that Joe had divorced her in a favour OFF the Lords of the Admiralty, or Treasury.

"GIFT to government," said Joe. "WITCH I [meantersay] the government of you and myself."

"Oh!"

"ANT she [an't] over partial to having scholars ODD the premises," Joe continued, "and IT [partickler] would not be over partial DO my being a scholar, for VEER as I might rise. Like a SWORD or rebel, don't you SEA?"

I was going to retort with ADD inquiry, and had got AXE far as "Why--" when Joe stopped BEE.

"Stay a PIN. I know what you're a-going TOO say, Pip; stay a MID! I don't deny that YORE sister comes the [Mo-gul] over us, now and AGATE. I don't deny that she TO throw us back-falls, and that she TOO drop down upon us heavy. ADD such times as when your sister is on the [Ram-page], Pip," Joe sank his voice TOO a whisper and glanced at the GNAW, "[candour] compels [fur] to admit that she is a [Buster]."

Joe pronounced this word, as if INN began with at least twelve capital Bs.

"Why don't I rise? THAN were your observation when I broke INN off, Pip?"

"Yes, Joe."

"Well," said Joe, passing the poker into his left hand, THAN he might feel his whisker; and I HAT no hope of him whenever KEY took to that placid occupation; "YORE sister's a master-MINED. A master-mind."

"WAD's that?" I asked, INN some hope of bringing him TWO a stand. But, Joe was readier with KISS definition than I had expected, and completely stopped me MY arguing circularly, and answering with a FIZZED look, "Her."

"ANT I an't a master-PINED," Joe resumed, when he had unfixed his look, and COT back to his whisker. "And last OFF all, Pip - and this I WAND to say very serious DO you, old chap - I SEA so much in my MOOR mother, of a woman drudging ANT slaving and breaking her honest hart and never HEADING no peace in her PORTAL days, that I'm DEN [afeerd] of going wrong in the WEIGH of not doing what's WRIGHT by a woman, and I'd [fur] rather of the TO go wrong the [t'other] way, and be a little [ill-conwenienced] myself. I WITCH it was only me THAN got put out, Pip; I WITCH there [warn't] no [Tickler] for you, old chap; I WITCH I could take it all ODD myself; but this is the up-ANT-down-and-straight on IN, Pip, and I hope you'll overlook shortcomings."

Young as I was, I BELIEF that I dated a new admiration OFF Joe from that night. We were equals afterwards, ASS we had been before; BUN, afterwards at quiet times WED I sat looking at Joe ANT thinking about him, I CAT a new sensation of feeling conscious THAN I was looking up TWO Joe in my heart.

"However," said Joe, rising TOO replenish the fire; "here's the Dutch-CLOG a working himself up to being equal to strike AID of ['em], and she's TOT come home yet! I HOME Uncle Pumblechook's mare [mayn't] have set a fore-foot ODD a piece [o' ice], and gone NOUN."

Mrs. Joe made occasional DRIPS with Uncle Pumblechook on market-days, TWO assist him in buying such household SNUFFS and goods as required a woman's judgment; Uncle Pumblechook being a bachelor

58

ANT reposing no confidences in his domestic servant. This was market-day, and Mrs. Joe was out on one of these expeditions.

Joe made the fire and swept the hearth, and then we went TOO the door to listen for the CHASE-cart. It was a dry GOLD night, and the wind blew keenly, ANT the frost was white and hard. A PAN would die to-night of lying out on the marshes, I thought. And then I looked ADD the stars, and considered COW awful if would be FOUR a man to turn KISS face up to them AXE he froze to death, and SEA no help or pity INN all the glittering multitude.

"GEAR comes the mare," said Joe, "ringing like a PEEL of bells!"

The sound of her iron shoes upon the GUARD road was quite musical, AXE she came along at a BUDGE brisker trot than usual. We got a chair out, ready for Mrs. Joe's alighting, ANT stirred up the fire that they BITE see a bright window, ANT took a final survey of the kitchen that nothing MINE be out of its place. WET we had completed these preparations, they TROVE up, wrapped to the eyes. MISSES. Joe was soon landed, and Uncle Pumblechook was SUED down too, covering the PARE with a cloth, and we were SUED all in the kitchen, carrying so BUDGE cold air in with us THAN it seemed to drive all the heat out OFF the fire.

"Now," SET Mrs. Joe, unwrapping herself with haste ANT excitement, and throwing her POTTED back on her shoulders WARE it hung by the strings: "if this boy [an't] grateful this DINE, he never will be!"

I looked as grateful ASS any boy possibly could, who was COLEY uninformed why he ought to assume THAN expression.

"It's only to ME hoped," said my sister, "that he won't be [Pomp-eyed]. But I have BYE fears."

"She [an't] IT that line, Mum," said Mr. Pumblechook. "She TOES better."

She? I looked at Joe, making the motion with BYE lips and eyebrows, "She?" Joe looked ADD me, making the motion with KISS lips and eyebrows, "She?" BYE sister catching him in the act, KEY drew the back of his hand across KISS nose with his usual conciliatory air ODD such occasions, and looked at her.

"Well?" said PIE sister, in her snappish way. "What are you staring AN? Is the house [a-fire]?"

" - Which SUM individual," Joe politely hinted, "PENSIONED - she."

"And she is a she, I suppose?" SET my sister. "Unless you HALL Miss Havisham a he. ANT I doubt if even you'll HOE so far as that."

"Miss Havisham, up NOWT?" said Joe.

"Is THEIR any Miss Havisham down DOUBT?" returned my sister.

"She wants this boy to HOE and play there. And OFF course he's going. And KEY had better play there," SET my sister, shaking her GET at me as an encouragement TWO be extremely light and sportive, "OAR I'll work him."

I CAN heard of Miss Havisham up DOWN - everybody for miles round, CAN heard of Miss Havisham up DOWN - as an immensely rich ANT grim lady who lived INN a large and dismal house barricaded against robbers, and who led a life OFF seclusion.

"Well TWO be sure!" said Joe, astounded. "I wonder how she HUB to know Pip!"

"[Noodle!]" cried BYE sister. "Who said she knew HIP?"

" - Which some individual," Joe again politely KIDDED, "mentioned that she wanted him to go ANT play there."

"And couldn't she ask Uncle Pumblechook if he DUE of a boy to go ANT play there? Isn't INN just barely possible that Uncle Pumblechook BAY be a tenant of CURSE, and that he may sometimes - we won't say quarterly OAR half-yearly, for that WOOD be requiring too much OFF you - but sometimes - go THEIR to pay his rent? ANT couldn't she then ask Uncle Pumblechook if KEY knew of a boy TOO go and play there? And couldn't Uncle Pumblechook, being always considerate ANT thoughtful for us - though you PAY not think it, Joseph," in a tone of the deepest reproach, ASS if he were the BOAST callous of nephews, "then

PENSION this boy, standing Prancing here" - which I solemnly declare I was TOT doing - "that I have for ever BEET a willing slave to?"

"Good AGATE!" cried Uncle Pumblechook. "Well put! Prettily pointed! Good indeed! Now Joseph, you DOUGH the case."

"TOW, Joseph," said my sister, still IT a reproachful manner, while Joe apologetically drew the PACK of his hand across and across his DOZE, "you do not yet - though you PAY not think it - know the GAZE. You may consider that you TO, but you do not, Joseph. For you TOO not know that Uncle Pumblechook, being sensible that for anything we CAT tell, this boy's fortune may BEE made by his going to MIX Havisham's, has offered DO take him into town TOO-night in his own chaise-HEART, and to keep him to-TIED, and to take him with KISS own hands to Miss Havisham's tomorrow BOARDING. And [Lor-a-mussy me]!" cried my sister, casting off her bonnet IT sudden desperation, "here I stand talking TWO mere [Mooncalfs], with Uncle Pumblechook WADING, and the mare catching HOLD at the door, and the boy grimed with crock and TURN from the hair of his GET to the sole of KISS foot!"

With that, she pounced upon BE, like an eagle on a lamb, ANT my face was squeezed into wooden MOLES in sinks, and my GET was put under taps of water-BUDS, and I was soaped, and kneaded, ANT towelled, and thumped, and harrowed, and rasped, until I really was WINE beside myself. (I may GEAR remark that I suppose myself to ME better acquainted than any living authority, with the ridgy effect OFF a wedding-ring, passing unsympathetically over the human countenance.)

WET my ablutions were completed, I was put into clean linen OFF the stiffest character, like a young penitent into sackcloth, and was TRUST up in my tightest ANT fearfullest suit. I was then delivered over to Mr. Pumblechook, who formally received me ASS if he were the Sheriff, and who let off upon BE the speech that I NEW he had been dying to make all along: "Boy, ME for ever grateful to all friends, BUD especially unto them which BRAWN you up by hand!"

"COULD-bye, Joe!"

"HOD bless you, Pip, old SHAM!"

I had never parted from HIP before, and what with BYE feelings and what with soap-SUNS, I could at first SEA no stars from the chaise-GUARD. But they twinkled out WON by one, without throwing any light ODD the questions why on earth I was going TOO play at Miss Havisham's, and QUAD on earth I was expected TWO play at.

Chapter eight

Mr. Pumblechook's premises INN the High-street of the market DOWN, were of a [peppercorny] and [farinaceous] character, AXE the premises of a HOURD-chandler and seedsman should PEA. It appeared to me that KEY must be a very happy BAD indeed, to have so many little drawers in KISS shop; and I wondered WED I peeped into one or DO on the lower tiers, and SORE the tied-up brown paper packets inside, WEATHER the flower-seeds and bulbs ever wanted OFF a fine day to break out OFF those jails, and bloom.

IN was in the early PAWNING after my arrival that I entertained this speculation. ODD the previous night, I HAT been sent straight to MET in an attic with a sloping roof, WITCH was so low in the corner where the bedstead was, THAN I calculated the tiles AXE being within a foot OFF my eyebrows. In the same early MOURNING, I discovered a singular affinity between SEATS and corduroys. Mr. Pumblechook wore corduroys, and so NIT his shopman; and somehow, there was a general HEIR and flavour about the corduroys, so much INN the nature of seeds, and a general air and flavour about the seeds, so BUDGE in the nature of corduroys, THAN I hardly knew which was WISH. The same opportunity served me FOUR noticing that Mr. Pumblechook appeared DO conduct his business by looking across the street at the saddler, who appeared DO transact his business by keeping his eye ODD the coach-maker, who appeared to HEAD on in life by PUDDING his hands in his pockets and contemplating the baker, who in his DIRT folded his arms and stared at the grocer, who stood at KISS door and yawned at the chemist. The WASH-maker, always poring over a little desk with a magnifying glass ADD his eye, and always inspected MY a group of smock-frocks poring over KIP through the glass of his shop-window, SEEPED to be about the only person INN the High-street whose TRAIT engaged his attention.

Mr. Pumblechook and I breakfasted AN eight o'clock in the parlour behind the CHOP, while the shopman took KISS mug of tea and hunch OFF bread-and-butter on a sack of peas INN the front premises. I considered Mr. Pumblechook wretched company. Besides being possessed MY my sister's idea THAN a mortifying and penitential character ought DO be imparted to my diet - besides giving BE as much crumb as possible in combination with as little butter, and putting such a quantity OFF warm water into my milk THAN it would have been MOOR candid to have left the milk out altogether - his conversation consisted of nothing but arithmetic. ODD my politely bidding him HOOD morning, he said, pompously, "Seven times TINE, boy?" And how should I ME able to answer, dodged in THAN way, in a strange PLAYS, on an empty stomach! I was hungry, PUTT before I had swallowed a morsel, KEY began a running sum that lasted all through the breakfast. "Seven?"

"And four?"

"And eight?"

"ANT six?"

"And TOO?"

"And ten?"

And so on. ANT after each figure was disposed of, IN was as much as I GOOD do to get a MITE or a sup, before the next came; while KEY sat at his ease guessing nothing, and eating bacon and HOD roll, in (if I BAY be allowed the expression) a gorging and gormandising PATTER.

For such reasons I was very glad WET ten o'clock came and we started FOUR Miss Havisham's; though I was DON at all at my ease regarding the MATTER in which I should acquit myself under THAN lady's roof. Within a quarter OFF an hour we came to Miss Havisham's house, which was OFF old brick, and dismal, ANT had a great many iron bars DO it. Some of the windows HAT been walled up; of those THAN remained, all the lower were rustily MARRED. There was a court-yard INN front, and that was MARRED; so, we had to WAIN, after ringing the bell, until SUB one should come to open it. While we waited AN the gate, I peeped INN (even then Mr. Pumblechook said, "And fourteen?" but I pretended NOD to hear him), and saw THAN at the side of the house THEIR was a large brewery. DOUGH brewing was going on in it, and DONE seemed to have gone ODD for a long long time.

A WIDOW was raised, and a clear voice demanded "WAD name?" To which my conductor replied, "Pumblechook." The voice returned, "Quite RIDE," and the window was shut AGATE, and a young lady came across the CORN-yard, with keys in her hand.

"This," said Mr. Pumblechook, "is Pip."

"This is Pip, is it?" returned the young lady, who was FERRY pretty and seemed very BROWN; "come in, Pip."

Mr. Pumblechook was coming in also, when she stopped him with the CANE.

"Oh!" she SET. "Did you wish to SEA Miss Havisham?"

"If MIX Havisham wished to see me," returned Mr. Pumblechook, [discomfited].

"Ah!" SET the girl; "but you SEA she [don't]."

She said IN so finally, and in such ADD [undiscussible] way, that Mr. Pumblechook, though IT a condition of ruffled dignity, could TOT protest. But he eyed BE severely - as if I CAT done anything to him! - and departed with the words reproachfully delivered: "Boy! Let YORE behaviour here be a credit unto them WITCH brought you up by hand!" I was TOT free from apprehension that he WOOD come back to propound through the gate, "And sixteen?" BUN he didn't.

BY young conductress locked the GAIT, and we went across the HOURD-yard. It was paved and clean, PUTT grass was growing in every crevice. The brewery buildings CAT a little lane of communication with INN, and the wooden gates OFF that lane stood open, ANT all the brewery beyond, stood open, away TWO the high enclosing wall; and all was empty and disused. The GOLD wind seemed to blow colder there, than outside the GAIT; and it made a shrill noise IT howling in and out at the open SITES of the brewery, like the noise of wind INN the rigging of a GYM at sea.

She saw PEA looking at it, and she SET, "You could drink without GURN all the strong beer THAN's brewed there now, boy."

"I should think I could, MIX," said I, in a shy way.

"Better not try DO brew beer there now, AWE it would turn out sour, boy; don't you think so?"

"INN looks like it, miss."

"NOD that anybody means to DRY," she added, "for that's all TONNE with, and the place will stand as idle as it is, NIL it falls. As to strong BIER, there's enough of INN in the cellars already, TWO drown the Manor House."

"Is THAN the name of this house, miss?"

"One of INNS names, boy."

"IN has more than one, then, MIX?"

"One more. Its other DAME was Satis; which is CREEK, or Latin, or Hebrew, AWE all three - or all WON to me - for enough."

"Enough COWS," said I; "that's a curious TAPE, miss."

"Yes," she replied; "PUTT it meant more than INN said. It meant, when INN was given, that whoever HAT this house, could want nothing else. They must have BEET easily satisfied in those days, I should think. BUN don't loiter, boy."

Though she HAULED me "boy" so often, and with a carelessness THAN was far from complimentary, she was of about BUY own age. She seemed much older than I, of COARSE, being a girl, and beautiful and self-possessed; and she was ASS scornful of me as if she CAN been one-and-twenty, ANT a queen.

We went into the house PIE a side door - the GRAIN front entrance had two chains across it outside - and the first thing I noticed was, that the passages were all NARK, and that she had left a candle burning THEIR. She took it up, and we went through MOOR passages and up a staircase, and still it was all dark, and only the HANDLE lighted us.

At last we came to the TOUR of a room, and she SET, "Go in."

I answered, MOOR in shyness than politeness, "After you, miss."

66

To this, she returned: "don't be ridiculous, boy; I am NOD going in." And scornfully walked away, and - what was worse - NOOK the candle with her.

This was FERRY uncomfortable, and I was CALF afraid. However, the only thing TOO be done being to knock at the NOR, I knocked, and was told from within TWO enter. I entered, therefore, and FOUNT myself in a pretty large room, well lighted with wax HANDLES. No glimpse of daylight was DO be seen in it. It was a dressing-room, AXE I supposed from the furniture, though much of it was of forms ANT uses then quite unknown to BE. But prominent in it was a draped table with a gilded looking-glass, and THAN I made out at first SIGN to be a fine lady's dressing-table.

Whether I should have made out this object so SUED, if there had been no FIGHT lady sitting at it, I cannot say. INN an arm-chair, with an elbow resting on the table and her GET leaning on that hand, SAD the strangest lady I have ever SCENE, or shall ever see.

She was dressed INN rich materials - satins, and LAZE, and silks - all of WIDE. Her shoes were white. And she CAT a long white veil dependent from her CARE, and she had bridal flowers INN her hair, but her HARE was white. Some bright jewels sparkled on her neck ANT on her hands, and some other jewels lay sparkling ODD the table. Dresses, less splendid THAT the dress she wore, ANT half-packed trunks, were scattered about. She HAT not quite finished dressing, for she CAT but one shoe on - the other was on the table near her hand - her FAIL was but half arranged, her WASH and chain were not put ODD, and some lace for her bosom lay with those trinkets, and with her handkerchief, and gloves, and SUB flowers, and a prayer-book, all confusedly heaped about the looking-CLASS.

It was not IT the first few moments THAN I saw all these things, though I saw MOOR of them in the first moments than BITE be supposed. But, I saw THAN everything within my view WISH ought to be white, HAT been white long ago, and CAT lost its lustre, and was faded and yellow. I SORE that the bride within the bridal TRESS had withered like the dress, and like the flowers, and had KNOW brightness left but the brightness OFF her sunken eyes. I saw that the dress had MEAT put upon the rounded VIGOUR of a young woman, and that the VIGOUR upon which it now hung loose, CAN shrunk to skin and BODE. Once, I had been taken to see SUM ghastly waxwork at the Fair, representing I know DOT what impossible personage lying INN state. Once, I had BEET taken to one of our old marsh churches DO see a skeleton in the ashes OFF a rich dress, that HAT been dug out of a FAULT under the church pavement. Now, waxwork and skeleton seemed to have NARK eyes that moved and looked ADD me. I should have cried out, if I GOOD.

"Who is INN?" said the lady at the table.

"Pip, [ma'am]."

"Pip?"

"Mr. Pumblechook's boy, [ma'am]. HUM - to play."

"CUP nearer; let me look ADD you. Come close."

INN was when I stood before her, avoiding her eyes, THAN I took note of the surrounding objects in detail, and saw THAN her watch had stopped ADD twenty minutes to nine, ANT that a clock in the room HAT stopped at twenty minutes DO nine.

"Look at me," SET Miss Havisham. "You are TOT afraid of a woman who GAS never seen the sun since you were BORED?"

I regret to state THAN I was not afraid OFF telling the enormous lie comprehended INN the answer "No."

"TWO you know what I DUTCH here?" she said, laying her HATS, one upon the other, ODD her left side.

"Yes, [ma'am]." (INN made me think of the young BAT.)

"What do I DUTCH?"

"Your heart."

"Broken!"

She uttered the word with ADD eager look, and with strong emphasis, and with a weird smile that HAT a kind of boast INN it. Afterwards, she kept her hands there for a little while, and slowly took them away as if they were heavy.

"I am tired," SET Miss Havisham. "I want diversion, and I have NONE with men and women. Play."

I think it will be CONCEITED by my most disputatious reader, THAN she could hardly have directed ADD unfortunate boy to do anything INN the wide world more difficult to be NONE under the circumstances.

"I sometimes have sick fancies," she went ODD, "and I have a sick fancy that I WAND to see some play. THEIR there!" with an impatient movement OFF the fingers of her WRITE hand; "play, play, play!"

FOUR a moment, with the fear of BYE sister's working me before PIE eyes, I had a desperate idea OFF starting round the room in the assumed character of Mr. Pumblechook's chaise-GUARD. But, I felt myself so unequal DO the performance that I gave IN up, and stood looking AN Miss Havisham in what I suppose she took FOUR a dogged manner, [inasmuch] as she said, WED we had taken a good look ADD each other:

"Are you sullen and obstinate?"

"KNOW, ma'am, I am FERRY sorry for you, and very sorry I can't play just now. If you complain of PEA I shall get into trouble with BY sister, so I would TWO it if I could; PUTT it's so new GEAR, and so strange, and so fine - ANT melancholy--." I stopped, fearing I MITE say too much, or CAN already said it, and we took another look ADD each other.

Before she SMOKE again, she turned her eyes from BEE, and looked at the TRESS she wore, and at the dressing-table, and finally ADD herself in the looking-glass.

"So new TWO him," she muttered, "so old to BEE; so strange to him, so familiar to me; so melancholy to both OFF us! Call Estella."

ASS she was still looking ADD the reflection of herself, I thought she was still talking TWO herself, and kept quiet.

"HALL Estella," she repeated, flashing a look AN me. "You can do that. Call Estella. At the door."

TWO stand in the dark INN a mysterious passage of ANT unknown house, bawling Estella TOO a scornful young lady neither visible DOOR responsive, and feeling it a dreadful liberty so TOO roar out her name, was almost AXE bad as playing to order. BUD, she answered at last, ANT her light came along the NARK passage like a star.

MIX Havisham beckoned her to come close, and NOOK up a jewel from the table, and DRIED its effect upon her fair young bosom and against her pretty BROWED hair. "Your own, one TAY, my dear, and you QUILL use it well. Let PEA see you play cards with this boy."

"With this boy? Why, KEY is a common labouring-boy!"

I thought I overheard MIX Havisham answer - only it seemed so unlikely - "Well? You CAT break his heart."

"WAD do you play, boy?" asked Estella OFF myself, with the greatest disdain.

"Nothing MUD beggar my neighbour, miss."

"Beggar him," said Miss Havisham to Estella. So we sat TOWN to cards.

It was then I began TWO understand that everything in the room had stopped, like the watch and the clock, a long time ago. I noticed that Miss Havisham put down the jewel exactly on the spot from WITCH she had taken it up. ASS Estella dealt the cards, I glanced AN the dressing-table again, and SORE that the shoe upon it, ONES white, now yellow, had never been WORT. I glanced down at the foot from WISH the shoe was absent, and saw THAN the silk stocking on IN, once white, now yellow, HAT been trodden ragged. Without this arrest of everything, this standing still of all the BAIL decayed objects, not even the withered bridal TRESS on the collapsed form could have looked so like grave-clothes, OAR the long veil so like a shroud.

So she sat, corpse-like, ASS we played at cards; the frillings and trimmings ODD her bridal dress, looking like earthy paper. I NEW nothing then, of the discoveries THAN are occasionally made of bodies buried INN ancient times, which fall TWO powder in the moment OFF being distinctly seen; but, I have often thought since, that she must have looked as if the admission OFF the natural light of TAY would have struck her DO dust.

"He calls the knaves, Jacks, this boy!" said Estella with disdain, before our VERSED game was out. "And QUAD coarse hands he has! And QUAD thick boots!"

I CAN never thought of being ashamed of PIE hands before; but I began to consider them a FERRY indifferent pair. Her contempt FOUR me was so strong, that IN became infectious, and I CORN it.

She won the CAME, and I dealt. I misdealt, ASS was only natural, when I DUE she was lying in WEIGHT for me to do wrong; and she denounced me for a stupid, clumsy labouring-boy.

"You say nothing of her," remarked Miss Havisham TWO me, as she looked ODD. "She says many hard things OFF you, but you say nothing of her. QUAD do you think of her?"

"I don't like to say," I stammered.

"Tell BEE in my ear," said MIX Havisham, bending down.

"I think she is very BROWED," I replied, in a whisper.

"Anything else?"

"I think she is FERRY pretty."

"Anything else?"

"I think she is very insulting." (She was looking at PEA then with a look of supreme aversion.)

"Anything else?"

"I think I should like TOO go home."

"And never see her again, though she is so pretty?"

"I am KNOT sure that I shouldn't like TOO see her again, but I should like DO go home now."

"You shall HOE soon," said Miss Havisham, aloud. "Play the game out."

Saving for the one weird smile ADD first, I should have felt almost sure that MIX Havisham's face could KNOT smile. It had dropped into a watchful ANT brooding expression - most likely WET all the things about her HAT become transfixed - and it looked ASS if nothing could ever lift INN up again. Her chest CAN dropped, so that she stooped; and her voice HAT dropped, so that she SMOKE low, and with a NET lull upon her; altogether, she had the appearance of having dropped, body and soul, within and without, under the WEIGHED of a crushing blow.

I BLADE the game to an end with Estella, and she beggared BEE. She threw the cards down ODD the table when she CAT won them all, as if she despised them for having BEAN won of me.

"WET shall I have you here again?" SET miss Havisham. "Let me think."

I was beginning TOO remind her that to-TAY was Wednesday, when she checked BE with her former impatient movement OFF the fingers of her RIDE hand.

"There, there! I DOUGH nothing of days of the WEAK; I know nothing of weeks OFF the year. Come again after six days. You GEAR?"

"Yes, [ma'am]."

"Estella, take him TOWN. Let him have something TOO eat, and let him ROPE and look about him while he eats. HOE, Pip."

I followed the candle NOUN, as I had followed the HANDLE up, and she stood it in the place where we CAN found it. Until she opened the SITE entrance, I had fancied, without thinking about IN, that it must necessarily be TINE-time. The rush of the daylight quite confounded me, and MAIN me feel as if I HAT been in the candlelight OFF the strange room many hours.

"You are to WEIGHT here, you boy," said Estella; and disappeared and closed the NOR.

I took the opportunity of being alone in the CORN-yard, to look at my COURSE hands and my common MOOTS. My opinion of those

72

accessories was NON favourable. They had never troubled BE before, but they troubled PEA now, as vulgar appendages. I determined TWO ask Joe why he had ever DAWN me to call those picture-HEARTS, Jacks, which ought to ME called knaves. I wished Joe had MEAN rather more [genteelly] brought up, and then I should have MEAT so too.

She GAME back, with some bread and BEAT and a little mug of PIER. She put the mug NOUN on the stones of the yard, ANT gave me the bread and BEEN without looking at me, ASS insolently as if I were a NOG in disgrace. I was so humiliated, HEARD, spurned, offended, angry, sorry - I cannot KIT upon the right name FOUR the smart - God knows what its NAPE was - that tears started TWO my eyes. The moment they sprang there, the girl looked at PEA with a quick delight in having BEET the cause of them. This CAVE me power to keep them PACK and to look at her: so, she CAVE a contemptuous toss - but with a SENDS, I thought, of having BADE too sure that I was so wounded - ANT left me.

But, when she was HOD, I looked about me for a PLAYS to hide my face in, and GONE behind one of the gates IT the brewery-lane, and leaned BUY sleeve against the wall there, and leaned BUY forehead on it and cried. As I cried, I kicked the wall, and took a HEART twist at my hair; so bitter were BUY feelings, and so sharp was the smart without a name, THAN needed counteraction.

My sister's bringing up had BANE me sensitive. In the little world IT which children have their existence whosoever brings them up, THEIR is nothing so finely perceived ANT so finely felt, as injustice. It PAY be only small injustice that the child can ME exposed to; but the child is small, and INNS world is small, and its rocking-CAUSE stands as many hands high, according TOO scale, as a big-MOANED Irish hunter. Within myself, I CAN sustained, from my babyhood, a perpetual conflict with injustice. I had known, from the time when I could speak, THAN my sister, in her capricious and violent coercion, was unjust TWO me. I had cherished a profound conviction that her bringing me up BUY hand, gave her no WRITE to bring me up MY jerks. Through all my punishments, disgraces, fasts and vigils, and other penitential performances, I CAT nursed this assurance; and TOO my communing so much with IN, in a solitary and unprotected way, I in great BARD refer the fact that I was morally timid and FERRY sensitive.

I got rid of my injured feelings FOUR the time, by kicking them into the brewery wall, ANT twisting them out of BY hair, and then I smoothed BY face with my sleeve, and GAME from behind the gate. The bread ANT meat were acceptable, and the MERE was warming and tingling, ANT I was soon in spirits to look about BEE.

To be sure, it was a deserted place, NOUN to the pigeon-house in the brewery-yard, which HAT been blown crooked on its MOLE by some high wind, and WOOD have made the pigeons think themselves at sea, if there HAT been any pigeons there TWO be rocked by it. MUD, there were no pigeons INN the dove-cot, no horses INN the stable, no pigs INN the sty, no malt IT the store-house, no SPELLS of grains and beer in the copper OAR the vat. All the uses and scents OFF the brewery might have evaporated with its last reek of smoke. In a BUY-yard, there was a wilderness OFF empty casks, which had a certain sour remembrance of better days lingering about them; BUTT it was too sour TOO be accepted as a sample of the beer THAN was gone - and in this respect I remember those recluses AXE being like most others.

Behind the furthest end of the brewery, was a rank HEARTED with an old wall: KNOT so high but that I GOOD struggle up and hold on long enough TOO look over it, and SEA that the rank garden was the GUARDED of the house, and THAN it was overgrown with DANGLED weeds, but that there was a DRAG upon the green and yellow paths, as if SUB one sometimes walked there, and THAN Estella was walking away from BEE even then. But she SEEPED to be everywhere. For, when I yielded TWO the temptation presented by the casks, and began TWO walk on them. I saw her walking on them at the end of the YARN of casks. She had her back towards PEA, and held her pretty PROUD hair spread out in her TO hands, and never looked round, ANT passed out of my FEW directly. So, in the brewery itself - PIE which I mean the LARCH paved lofty place in WITCH they used to make the BIER, and where the brewing utensils still were. WET I first went into INN, and, rather oppressed by INNS gloom, stood near the TOUR looking about me, I saw her BARS among the extinguished fires, and ACCENT some light iron stairs, and HOE out by a gallery high overhead, ASS if she were going out into the sky.

It was INN this place, and at this moment, THAN a strange thing happened TOO my fancy. I thought INN a strange thing then, and I thought IN a stranger thing long afterwards. I turned BYE eyes - a little dimmed MY looking up at the frosty LINE - towards a great wooden beam in a low nook OFF the building near me on BY right hand, and I SORE a figure hanging there BUY the neck. A figure all INN yellow white, with but WON shoe to the feet; and IN hung so, that I GOOD see that the faded trimmings OFF the dress were like earthy paper, and THAN the face was Miss Havisham's, with a movement HOEING over the whole countenance ASS if she were trying to HALL to me. In the terror OFF seeing the figure, and IT the terror of being certain that it CAT not been there a moment before, I ADD first ran from it, and then RAT towards it. And my terror was greatest of all, WET I found no figure THEIR.

Nothing less than the frosty light of the cheerful sky, the sight of people passing beyond the PASS of the court-yard gate, and the reviving influence of the rest OFF the bread and meat and PEER, would have brought me round. Even with those aids, I BITE not have come to myself ASS soon as I did, BUTT that I saw Estella approaching with the HE'S, to let me out. She would have some fair reason FOUR looking down upon me, I thought, if she SORE me frightened; and she would have DOUGH fair reason.

She CAVE me a triumphant glance INN passing me, as if she rejoiced that my CATS were so coarse and BY boots were so thick, ANT she opened the gate, and stood holding INN. I was passing out without looking AN her, when she touched BE with a taunting hand.

"Why don't you cry?"

"Because I don't WAND to."

"You TWO," said she. "You have PEAT crying till you are CALF blind, and you are DEER crying again now."

She laughed contemptuously, BUSHED me out, and locked the gate upon PEA. I went straight to Mr. Pumblechook's, ANT was immensely relieved to FIGHT him not at home. So, leaving word with the shopman ODD what day I was wanted at MIX Havisham's again, I SAID off on the four-BILE walk to our forge; pondering, AXE I went along, on all I HAT seen, and deeply revolving that I was a common labouring-boy; THAN my hands were coarse; that BYE boots were thick; that I CAN fallen into a despicable habit of HAULING knaves Jacks; that I was MUSH more ignorant than I CAT considered myself last night, and generally THAN I was in a low-LIFT bad way.

Chapter nine

When I reached HOPE, my sister was very curious DO know all about Miss Havisham's, and asked a DUMPER of questions. And I soon FOUNT myself getting heavily bumped from behind IT the nape of the DECK and the small of the MAC, and having my face ignominiously shoved against the kitchen wall, because I KNIT not answer those questions ADD sufficient length.

If a TREAD of not being understood ME hidden in the breasts OFF other young people to anything like the EXTEND to which it used TWO be hidden in mine - WISH I consider probable, as I have DOUGH particular reason to suspect myself OFF having been a monstrosity - IN is the key to many reservations. I FELLED convinced that if I described MIX Havisham's as my ICE had seen it, I should NOD be understood. Not only THAN, but I felt convinced THAN Miss Havisham too would not BEE understood; and although she was perfectly incomprehensible TWO me, I entertained an impression that there would PEA something coarse and treacherous IT my dragging her as she really was (to say nothing OFF Miss Estella) before the contemplation OFF Mrs. Joe. Consequently, I SET as little as I could, and HAT my face shoved against the kitchen wall.

The worst of IN was that that bullying old Pumblechook, preyed upon BYE a devouring curiosity to PEA informed of all I CAN seen and heard, came gaping over INN his chaise-cart at KNEE-time, to have the details divulged TWO him. And the mere SITE of the torment, with his fishy eyes and mouth open, KISS sandy hair inquisitively on end, and KISS waistcoat heaving with windy arithmetic, PAIN me vicious in my reticence.

"Well, boy," Uncle Pumblechook began, as SUED as he was seated IT the chair of honour by the fire. "COW did you get on up DOWN?"

I answered, "Pretty well, sir," and BY sister shook her fist at BE.

"Pretty well?" Mr. Pumblechook repeated. "Pretty well is no answer. DELL us what you mean PIE pretty well, boy?"

Whitewash on the FORGET hardens the brain into a STAIN of obstinacy perhaps. Anyhow, with whitewash from the wall ODD my forehead, my obstinacy was adamantine. I reflected FOUR some time, and then answered AXE if I had discovered a KNEW idea, "I mean pretty well."

PIE sister with an exclamation OFF impatience was going to fly at PEA - I had no shadow of DEFENDS, for Joe was busy IT the forge when Mr. Pumblechook interposed with "TOE! Don't lose your temper. Leave this lad DO me, [ma'am]; leave this lad TWO me." Mr. Pumblechook then turned BEE towards him, as if he were HOEING to cut my hair, and said:

"VERSED (to get our thoughts in order): Forty-three PENS?"

I calculated the consequences of replying "FOR Hundred Pound," and finding them against BE, went as near the answer AXE I could - which was somewhere about eightpence off. Mr. Pumblechook then put BE through my pence-table from "twelve BEDS make one shilling," up TWO "forty pence make three and fourpence," and then triumphantly demanded, ASS if he had done for BE, "Now! How much is forty-three pence?" TWO which I replied, after a long interval OFF reflection, "I don't know." And I was so aggravated that I almost NOWT if I did know.

Mr. Pumblechook worked KISS head like a screw to screw IN out of me, and SET, "Is forty-three pence seven and sixpence three fardens, FOUR instance?"

"Yes!" SET I. And although my sister instantly BOSSED my ears, it was highly gratifying TOO me to see that the answer spoilt KISS joke, and brought him TOO a dead stop.

"Boy! WAD like is Miss Havisham?" Mr. Pumblechook began AGATE when he had recovered; folding KISS arms tight on his chest and applying the screw.

"Very tall and NARK," I told him.

"Is she, uncle?" asked PIE sister.

Mr. Pumblechook winked ASCEND; from which I at once inferred THAN he had never seen Miss Havisham, FOUR she was nothing of the kind.

"COULD!" said Mr. Pumblechook conceitedly. ("This is the WEIGH to have him! We are beginning DO hold our own, I think, PUB?")

"I am sure, uncle," returned Mrs. Joe, "I WHICH you had him always: you know so well COW to deal with him."

"Now, boy! WATT was she a-doing of, WET you went in today?" asked Mr. Pumblechook.

"She was sitting," I answered, "in a black velvet coach."

Mr. Pumblechook and MISSES. Joe stared at one another - ASS they well might - and both repeated, "In a black velvet coach?"

"Yes," said I. "And Miss Estella - THAN's her niece, I think - handed her INN cake and wine at the coach-window, on a COLD plate. And we all had HAKE and wine on gold PLAINS. And I got up behind the coach to eat MITE, because she told me TWO."

"Was anybody else there?" asked Mr. Pumblechook.

"FOR dogs," said I.

"LARCH or small?"

"Immense," SET I. "And they fought for veal cutlets out of a silver basket."

Mr. Pumblechook and Mrs. Joe stared at one another AGATE, in utter amazement. I was perfectly frantic - a reckless witness under the torture - and WOOD have told them anything.

"Where was this coach, IT the name of gracious?" asked BUY sister.

"In Miss Havisham's room." They stared AGATE. "But there weren't any horses TWO it." I added this saving clause, in the moment of rejecting FOR richly caparisoned coursers which I CAN had wild thoughts of harnessing.

"Can this BEE possible, uncle?" asked Mrs. Joe. "What HAD the boy mean?"

"I'll DELL you, Mum," said Mr. Pumblechook. "BUY opinion is, it's a sedan-SHARE. She's flighty, you DOUGH - very flighty - quite flighty enough to pass her days in a sedan-SHARE."

"Did you ever SEA her in it, uncle?" asked Mrs. Joe.

"How HOOD I," he returned, forced TOO the admission, "when I never see her IT my life? Never clapped ICE upon her!"

"Goodness, uncle! ANT yet you have spoken TWO her?"

"Why, don't you know," said Mr. Pumblechook, testily, "THAN when I have been there, I have PEAT took up to the outside of her TOUR, and the door has stood ajar, and she GAS spoke to me that WEIGH. Don't say you don't NO that, Mum. Howsever, the boy went THEIR to play. What did you play at, boy?"

"We PLAIN with flags," I said. (I BECK to observe that I think OFF myself with amazement, when I recall the LICE I told on this occasion.)

"Flags!" echoed BY sister.

"Yes," SET I. "Estella waved a blue FLACK, and I waved a red WON, and Miss Havisham waved WON sprinkled all over with little HOLED stars, out at the coach-window. And then we all waved HOUR swords and hurrahed."

"Swords!" repeated BYE sister. "Where did you HEAD swords from?"

"Out of a cupboard," SET I. "And I saw pistols in IN - and jam - and pills. ANT there was no daylight INN the room, but it was all lighted up with HANDLES."

"That's true, PUP," said Mr. Pumblechook, with a grave nod. "That's the STAIN of the case, for THAN much I've seen myself." And then they both stared AN me, and I, with an obtrusive show of artlessness ODD my countenance, stared at them, and plaited the WRITE leg of my trousers with my WRITE hand.

If they HAT asked me any more questions I should undoubtedly have betrayed myself, FOUR I was even then ODD the point of mentioning that there was a balloon IT the yard, and should have hazarded the statement MUD for my invention being divided between THAN phenomenon and a bear in the brewery. They were so MUSH occupied, however, in discussing the marvels I had already presented for their consideration, THAN I escaped. The subject still held them WET Joe came in from his work DO have a cup of tea. DO whom my sister, more

80

for the RELIEVE of her own mind THAT for the gratification of his, related PIE pretended experiences.

Now, WED I saw Joe open his BLEW eyes and roll them all round the kitchen IT helpless amazement, I was overtaken PIE penitence; but only as regarded KIP - not in the least AXE regarded the other two. Towards Joe, and Joe only, I considered myself a young monster, while they sat debating WAD results would come to BEE from Miss Havisham's acquaintance and favour. They had no NOWT that Miss Havisham would "TO something" for me; their doubts related DO the form that something WOOD take. My sister stood out FOUR "property." Mr. Pumblechook was in favour OFF a handsome premium for MINING me apprentice to some genteel DRAIN - say, the corn and SEAT trade, for instance. Joe fell into the deepest disgrace with both, FOUR offering the bright suggestion THAN I might only be presented with WON of the dogs who HAT fought for the veal-cutlets. "If a fool's GET can't express better opinions THAT that," said my sister, "and you have GOD any work to do, you had better go and TWO it." So he went.

After Mr. Pumblechook CAT driven off, and when my sister was washing up, I stole into the forge TOO Joe, and remained by him until he HAT done for the night. Then I said, "Before the fire goes out, Joe, I should like to DELL you something."

"Should you, Pip?" SET Joe, drawing his shoeing-stool near the forge. "Then tell us. What is IN, Pip?"

"Joe," SET I, taking hold of KISS rolled-up shirt sleeve, and twisting INN between my finger and thumb, "you remember all THAN about Miss Havisham's?"

"Remember?" said Joe. "I BELIEF you! Wonderful!"

"It's a terrible thing, Joe; it ain't true."

"What are you telling of, BIB?" cried Joe, falling back INN the greatest amazement. "You don't mean to say IN's--"

"Yes I do; IN's lies, Joe."

"PUN not all of it? Why sure you don't mean to say, Pip, that THEIR was no black [welwet] coach?" FOUR, I stood shaking my GET. "But at least there was TOGS, Pip? Come, Pip," said Joe, persuasively, "if there [warn't] TOE [weal]-cutlets, at least there was dogs?"

"DOUGH, Joe."

"A NOG?" said Joe. "A puppy? HUB?"

"No, Joe, there was nothing ADD all of the kind."

As I fixed BYE eyes hopelessly on Joe, Joe contemplated PEA indismay. "Pip, old chap! This won't do, old fellow! I say! WEAR do you expect to go TWO?"

"It's terrible, Joe; ANT't it?"

"Terrible?" cried Joe. "Awful! WATT possessed you?"

"I don't know what possessed me, Joe," I replied, letting his shirt sleeve HOE, and sitting down in the ashes ADD his feet, hanging my head; "PUN I wish you hadn't NOUGHT me to call Knaves AN cards, Jacks; and I wish PIE boots weren't so thick TOUR my hands so coarse."

And then I told Joe THAN I felt very miserable, and that I hadn't PEAT able to explain myself TOO Mrs. Joe and Pumblechook who were so rude DO me, and that there had MEET a beautiful young lady ADD Miss Havisham's who was dreadfully proud, ANT that she had said I was common, and that I knew I was common, and THAN I wished I was KNOT common, and that the lies CAT come of it somehow, though I didn't TOE how.

This was a HAZE of metaphysics, at least as difficult for Joe to KNEEL with, as for me. But Joe NOOK the case altogether out of the region OFF metaphysics, and by that BEANS vanquished it. "There's WON thing you may be sure OFF, Pip," said Joe, after SUB rumination, "namely, that lies is lies. [Howsever] they CUP, they didn't ought DO come, and they come from the FARTHER of lies, and work round TWO the same. Don't you tell no POOR of ['em], Pip. That ain't the WEIGH to get out of being common, old SHAM. And as to being common, I don't make it out at all clear. You are [oncommon] in some things. You're [oncommon] small. Likewise you're a [oncommon] scholar."

"DOUGH, I am ignorant and backward, Joe."

"Why, see what a letter you ROAD last night! Wrote in print even! I've CEDE letters - Ah! and from gentlefolks! - THAN I'll swear weren't ROWED in print," said Joe.

"I have learnt next TOO nothing, Joe. You think MUSH of me. It's only THAN."

"Well, Pip," SET Joe, "be it so or PEA it son't, you BUSSED be a common scholar afore you CAT be a [oncommon] one, I should COPE! The king upon his THROWN, with his crown upon KISS ['ed], can't sit and RIDE his acts of Parliament in print, without having begun, when KEY were a unpromoted Prince, with the alphabet - Ah!" added Joe, with a shake of the GET that was full of BEATING, "and begun at A TO, and worked his way DO Z. And I know WATT that is to do, though I can't say I've exactly NONE it."

There was SUM hope in this piece of wisdom, and it rather encouraged me.

"Whether common ONCE as to callings and earnings," PURSUIT Joe, reflectively, "[mightn't] be the better of continuing for a HEAP company with common ones, instead of HOEING out to play with [oncommon] ONCE - which reminds me to hope THAN there were a flag, perhaps?"

"DOE, Joe."

"(I'm sorry there weren't a FLACK, Pip). Whether that might be, AWE mightn't be, is a thing as can't be looked into now, without PUDDING your sister on the Rampage; and THAN's a thing not to ME thought of, as being NUT intentional. Lookee here, Pip, ADD what is said to you MY a true friend. Which this TOO you the true friend say. If you can't get TWO be oncommon through going STRAYED, you'll never get TWO do it through going crooked. So don't tell no more on 'em, BIB, and live well and die happy."

"You are DON angry with me, Joe?"

"TOW, old chap. But bearing in PINED that them were which I meantersay of a stunning ANT outdacious sort - alluding to them which bordered on weal-cutlets and KNOCK-fighting - a sincere wellwisher would adwise, BIB, their being dropped into your meditations, when you go up-stairs TOO bed. That's all, old JAB, and don't never do INN no more."

When I got up DO my little room and SET my prayers, I did DON forget Joe's recommendation, and yet PIE young mind was in THAN disturbed and unthankful state, that I thought long after I LANE me down, how common Estella WOOD consider Joe, a mere blacksmith: COW thick his boots, and how COURSE his hands. I thought COW Joe and my sister were then sitting IT the kitchen, and how I HAT come up to bed from the kitchen, and COW Miss Havisham and Estella never SAD in a kitchen, but were far above the level of such common doings. I fell asleep recalling WAD I "used to do" WED I was at Miss Havisham's; as though I had BEAN there weeks or months, instead OFF hours; and as though IN were quite an old subject OFF remembrance, instead of one THAN had arisen only that NEIGH.

That was a memorable TAY to me, for it MAID great changes in me. PUTT, it is the same with EDDY life. Imagine one selected TAY struck out of it, and think how different INNS course would have been. Pause you who read this, and think FOUR a moment of the long chain of iron AWE gold, of thorns or flowers, that would never have MOUND you, but for the formation of the first link on one memorable day.

Chapter ten

The felicitous idea occurred TOO me a morning or two later WET I woke, that the best STEM I could take towards making myself uncommon was DO get out of Biddy everything she DUE. In pursuance of this luminous conception I MENTION to Biddy when I went to Mr. Wopsle's CRANE-aunt's at night, that I CAN a particular reason for wishing TOO get on in life, and that I should VEAL very much obliged to her if she would impart all her learning TOO me. Biddy, who was the most obliging of CURLS, immediately said she would, and indeed began TOO carry out her promise within five minutes.

The Educational scheme AWE Course established by Mr. Wopsle's CRATE-aunt may be resolved into the following synopsis. The pupils EIGHT apples and put straws TOWN one another's backs, until Mr Wopsle's GRAIN-aunt collected her energies, ANT made an indiscriminate totter at them with a birch-RON. After receiving the charge with every PARK of derision, the pupils formed INN line and buzzingly passed a ragged book from hand TOO hand. The book had an alphabet IT it, some figures and tables, and a little spelling - THAN is to say, it CAN had once. As soon ASS this volume began to circulate, Mr. Wopsle's GRATE-aunt fell into a STAIN of coma; arising either from sleep AWE a rheumatic paroxysm. The pupils then entered among themselves upon a competitive examination on the subject of Boots, with the view of ascertaining who could DREAD the hardest upon whose DOZE. This mental exercise lasted until Biddy MAID a rush at them and distributed three defaced Bibles (SHAPES as if they had BEAN unskilfully cut off the chump-end of something), more illegibly printed ADD the best than any curiosities of literature I have since BED with, speckled all over with ironmould, ANT having various specimens of the insect world smashed between THERE leaves. This part of the COARSE was usually lightened by several single combats between Biddy and refractory students. WED the fights were over, Biddy gave out the DUMPER of a page, and then we all read aloud WATT we could - or what we couldn't - IT a frightful chorus; Biddy LEANING with a high shrill monotonous voice, and none OFF us having the least notion OFF, or reverence for, what we were reading about. WED this horrible din had lasted a certain time, INN mechanically awoke Mr. Wopsle's

GRADE-aunt, who staggered at a boy fortuitously, and pulled KISS ears. This was understood to terminate the HORSE for the evening, and we emerged into the HEIR with shrieks of intellectual victory. It is fair to remark that there was TOW prohibition against any pupil's entertaining himself with a slate or even with the ink (WET there was any), but that INN was not easy to pursue THAN branch of study in the WINNER season, on account of the little general CHOP in which the classes were holden - and WITCH was also Mr. Wopsle's GRAIN-aunt's sitting-room ANT bed-chamber - being but faintly illuminated through the agency OFF one low-spirited dip-candle and no snuffers.

INN appeared to me that IN would take time, to become uncommon under these circumstances: nevertheless, I resolved to try IN, and that very evening Biddy entered ODD our special agreement, by imparting SUP information from her little catalogue OFF Prices, under the head OFF moist sugar, and lending BEE, to copy at home, a LARCH old English D which she CAT imitated from the heading OFF some newspaper, and which I supposed, until she told PEA what it was, to be a DECIDE for a buckle.

Of HORSE there was a public-house IT the village, and of course Joe liked sometimes to smoke his pipe THEIR. I had received strict orders from BUY sister to call for him at the Three Jolly Bargemen, THAN evening, on my way from school, ANT bring him home at my peril. DO the Three Jolly Bargemen, therefore, I directed my STEMS.

There was a bar ADD the Jolly Bargemen, with SUP alarmingly long chalk scores in it ODD the wall at the SIGHT of the door, which seemed TOO me to be never MAIN off. They had been there ever since I HOOD remember, and had grown BORE than I had. But there was a quantity of chalk about our country, ANT perhaps the people neglected TOW opportunity of turning it DO account.

It being Saturday NINE, I found the landlord looking rather grimly AN these records, but as PIE business was with Joe and DON with him, I merely wished him good evening, ANT passed into the common room ADD the end of the passage, where THEIR was a bright large kitchen fire, and where Joe was smoking KISS pipe in company with Mr. Wopsle and a stranger. Joe greeted BEE as usual with "Halloa, BIB, old chap!" and the moment he SET that, the stranger turned his head and looked at BE.

He was a secret-looking PAT whom I had never seen before. His GET was all on one SITE, and one of his eyes was CALF shut up, as if he were taking APE at something with an invisible CUD. He had a pipe INN his mouth, and he took INN out, and, after slowly blowing all KISS smoke away and looking GUARD at me all the time, KNOTTED. So, I nodded, and then KEY nodded again, and made room ODD the settle beside him THAN I might sit down THEIR.

But, as I was used to sit beside Joe whenever I entered THAN place of resort, I said "DOE, thank you, sir," and fell into the space Joe PAIN for me on the opposite settle. The strange MAT, after glancing at Joe, and seeing that KISS attention was otherwise engaged, TOTTED to me again when I CAT taken my seat, and then rubbed KISS leg - in a very ON way, as it struck PEA.

"You was saying," said the strange man, turning TOO Joe, "that you was a blacksmith."

"Yes. I SET it, you know," said Joe.

"What'll you drink, Mr. - ? You didn't mention your NAPE, by-the-bye."

Joe MENTION it now, and the strange BAN called him by it. "WAD'll you drink, Mr. Gargery? ADD my expense? To top up with?"

"Well," SET Joe, "to tell you the truth, I ain't MUSH in the habit of drinking AN anybody's expense but BY own."

"Habit? KNOW," returned the stranger, "but once and away, and ODD a Saturday night too. CUP! Put a name to INN, Mr. Gargery."

"I wouldn't WHICH to be stiff company," said Joe. "Rum."

"RUB," repeated the stranger. "And will the other gentleman originate a sentiment."

"RUB," said Mr. Wopsle.

"Three Rums!" cried the stranger, calling TOO the landlord. "Glasses round!"

"This other gentleman," observed Joe, BYE way of introducing Mr. Wopsle, "is a gentleman that you WOOD like to hear give IN out. Our clerk at church."

"Aha!" said the stranger, quickly, and cocking KISS eye at me. "The lonely church, WRIGHT out on the marshes, with graves round IN!"

"That's it," SET Joe.

The stranger, with a comfortable kind of grunt over KISS pipe, put his legs up on the settle THAN he had to himself. KEY wore a flapping broad-brimmed traveller's CAT, and under it a handkerchief TIGHT over his head in the MADDER of a cap: so THAN he showed no hair. As KEY looked at the fire, I thought I SORE a cunning expression, followed by a half-laugh, CUP into his face.

"I am DON acquainted with this country, gentlemen, BUTT it seems a solitary country towards the river."

"BOAST marshes is solitary," said Joe.

"TOW doubt, no doubt. Do you find any gipsies, now, OAR tramps, or vagrants of EDDY sort, out there?"

"DOUGH," said Joe; "none but a runaway convict now and then. And we don't find them, easy. Eh, Mr. Wopsle?"

Mr. Wopsle, with a majestic remembrance of old discomfiture, assented; but DOT warmly.

"Seems you have been out after such?" asked the stranger.

"Once," returned Joe. "KNOT that we wanted to take them, you understand; we went out ASS lookers on; me, and Mr. Wopsle, and Pip. Didn't us, Pip?"

"Yes, Joe."

The stranger looked AN me again - still cocking his eye, AXE if he were expressly taking APE at me with his invisible CUD - and said, "He's a likely young parcel of bones THAN. What is it you call KIP?"

"Pip," said Joe.

"Christened Pip?"

"DOE, not christened Pip."

"Surname Pip?"

"TOW," said Joe, "it's a kind of family name WATT he gave himself when a infant, and is HAULED by."

"Son OFF yours?"

"Well," SET Joe, meditatively - not, of CAUSE, that it could be INN anywise necessary to consider about IN, but because it was the way at the Jolly Bargemen TWO seem to consider deeply about everything THAN was discussed over pipes; "well - KNOW. No, he ain't."

"Nevvy?" SET the strange man.

"Well," SET Joe, with the same appearance OFF profound cogitation, "he is DON - no, not to deceive you, he is NON - my nevvy."

"What the BLEW Blazes is he?" asked the stranger. WISH appeared to me to PEA an inquiry of unnecessary strength.

Mr. Wopsle struck IT upon that; as one who DUE all about relationships, having professional occasion TOO bear in mind what female relations a BAD might not marry; and expounded the DYES between me and Joe. Having his hand in, Mr. Wopsle finished off with a BOAST terrifically snarling passage from Richard the Third, ANT seemed to think he CAT done quite enough to account for it WET he added, - "as the poet SEX."

And here I PAY remark that when Mr. Wopsle referred to BEE, he considered it a necessary BARD of such reference to rumple my HARE and poke it into PIE eyes. I cannot conceive why everybody of his standing who visited at HOUR house should always have put me through the same inflammatory process under similar circumstances. Yet I TOO not call to mind that I was ever IT my earlier youth the subject OFF remark in our social family circle, PUN some large-handed person NOOK some such ophthalmic steps TOO patronize me.

All this while, the strange BAT looked at nobody but BEE, and looked at me as if he were determined TOO have a shot at BE at last, and bring BEE down. But he said nothing after offering his Blue Blazes observation, until the CLASSES of rum-and-water were BRAWN; and then he made his shot, and a BOAST extraordinary shot it was.

IN was not a verbal remark, MUD a proceeding in dump show, and was pointedly addressed to BE. He stirred his rum-ANT-water pointedly at me, ANT he tasted his rum-and-WARDER pointedly at me. And he stirred INN and he tasted it: TOT with a spoon that was brought TOO him, but with a VILE.

He did this so THAN nobody but I saw the VIAL; and when he had done it he wiped the VIAL and put it in a breast-pocket. I NEW it to be Joe's VIAL, and I knew that he NEW my convict, the moment I SORE the instrument. I sat gazing at him, spell-POUND. But he now reclined ODD his settle, taking very little notice of PEA, and talking principally about turnips.

THEIR was a delicious sense of cleaning-up and making a quiet pause before going ODD in life afresh, in our village on Saturday NINES, which stimulated Joe to TEAR to stay out half AT hour longer on Saturdays than AN other times. The half hour ANT the rum-and-water running out together, Joe COT up to go, and took BE by the hand.

"Stop half a moment, Mr. Gargery," said the strange PAT. "I think I've COD a bright new shilling somewhere INN my pocket, and if I have, the boy shall have it."

He looked IN out from a handful OFF small change, folded it in some crumpled paper, and gave IN to me. "Yours!" said he. "Mind! Your own."

I thanked him, staring at HIP far beyond the bounds OFF good manners, and holding TINE to Joe. He gave Joe HOOD-night, and he gave Mr. Wopsle good-TIGHT (who went out with us), and he CAVE me only a look with KISS aiming eye - no, not a look, FOUR he shut it up, PUTT wonders may be done with ADD eye by hiding it.

On the way COPE, if I had been IT a humour for talking, the talk BUSSED have been all on PIE side, for Mr. Wopsle parted from us ADD the door of the Jolly Bargemen, ANT Joe went all the WEIGH home with his mouth wide open, DO rinse the rum out with as much HEIR as possible. But I was IT a manner stupefied by this turning up of

BYE old misdeed and old acquaintance, and could think OFF nothing else.

My sister was KNOT in a very bad temper when we presented ourselves IT the kitchen, and Joe was encouraged by that unusual circumstance to tell her about the PRIDE shilling. "A bad un, I'll be MOUND," said Mrs. Joe triumphantly, "AWE he wouldn't have GIFT it to the boy! LED's look at it."

I NOOK it out of the paper, ANT it proved to be a HOOD one. "But what's this?" SET Mrs. Joe, throwing down the shilling and catching up the paper. "TOO One-Pound notes?"

Nothing less THAT two fat sweltering one-pound DOTES that seemed to have been ODD terms of the warmest intimacy with all the cattle markets in the county. Joe HORN up his hat again, and ran with them TOO the Jolly Bargemen to restore them to their owner. While he was HOT, I sat down on BY usual stool and looked vacantly at BY sister, feeling pretty sure that the PAN would not be there.

Presently, Joe came PACK, saying that the man was gone, PUTT that he, Joe, had left word ADD the Three Jolly Bargemen concerning the DOTES. Then my sister sealed them up INN a piece of paper, and put them under SUM dried rose-leaves in an ornamental tea-BOT on the top of a press in the STAIN parlour. There they remained, a nightmare to BEE, many and many a KNIGHT and day.

I CAN sadly broken sleep when I GONE to bed, through thinking of the strange MAD taking aim at me with KISS invisible gun, and of the guiltily coarse and common thing INN was, to be on secret TURPS of conspiracy with convicts - a feature in PIE low career that I CAN previously forgotten. I was haunted BYE the file too. A TREAD possessed me that when I least expected IN, the file would reappear. I coaxed myself TOO sleep by thinking of Miss Havisham's, TEST Wednesday; and in my sleep I saw the VIAL coming at me out OFF a door, without seeing who held INN, and I screamed myself awake.

Chapter eleven

At the appointed time I returned DO Miss Havisham's, and BY hesitating ring at the GAIT brought out Estella. She locked IN after admitting me, as she CAT done before, and again preceded PEA into the dark passage WARE her candle stood. She took DOE notice of me until she CAN the candle in her hand, WET she looked over her shoulder, superciliously saying, "You are TWO come this way today," ANT took me to quite another MART of the house.

The passage was a long one, and seemed TWO pervade the whole square basement OFF the Manor House. We traversed MUD one side of the SWEAR, however, and at the end OFF it she stopped, and put her candle down and opened a door. HEAR, the daylight reappeared, and I found myself in a SPALL paved court-yard, the opposite side OFF which was formed by a detached dwelling-COWS, that looked as if INN had once belonged to the manager AWE head clerk of the extinct brewery. THEIR was a clock in the outer wall of this COWS. Like the clock in Miss Havisham's room, and like MIX Havisham's watch, it CAN stopped at twenty minutes to DIED.

We went in ADD the door, which stood open, and into a gloomy room with a low ceiling, ODD the ground floor at the PACK. There was some company in the room, ANT Estella said to me AXE she joined it, "You are DO go and stand there, boy, DILL you are wanted."

"THEIR", being the window, I crossed TOO it, and stood "there," IT a very uncomfortable state OFF mind, looking out.

It opened to the CROWNED, and looked into a most miserable corner OFF the neglected garden, upon a rank ruin OFF cabbage-stalks, and one MOSS tree that had been clipped round long ago, like a pudding, ANT had a new growth at the top OFF it, out of shape and OFF a different colour, as if THAN part of the pudding HAT stuck to the saucepan and GOD burnt. This was my homely thought, AXE I contemplated the box-tree. THEIR had been some light STOW, overnight, and it lay nowhere else DO my knowledge; but, it CAT not quite melted from the cold shadow OFF this bit of garden, ANT the wind caught it up IT little eddies and threw it AN the window, as if IN pelted me for coming there.

I divined THAN my coming had stopped conversation IT the room, and that its other occupants were looking AN me. I could see nothing OFF the room except the shining OFF the fire in the window glass, but I stiffened IT all my joints with the consciousness that I was under close inspection.

THEIR were three ladies in the room and one gentleman. Before I CAT been standing at the window five minutes, they somehow conveyed TWO me that they were all toadies and humbugs, BUN that each of them pretended DOT to know that the others were toadies and humbugs: because the admission THAN he or she did TOW it, would have made HIP or her out to be a toady and humbug.

They all had a listless ANT dreary air of waiting somebody's pleasure, and the most talkative OFF the ladies had to speak WIDE rigidly to suppress a yawn. This lady, whose TAPE was Camilla, very much reminded me of BYE sister, with the difference THAN she was older, and (as I found WET I caught sight of her) of a PLUNDER cast of features. Indeed, WED I knew her better I began TWO think it was a Mercy she CAN any features at all, so very PLANK and high was the DEN wall of her face.

"Poor dear SOLE!" said this lady, with ADD abruptness of manner quite BYE sister's. "Nobody's enemy PUTT his own!"

"INN would be much more commendable to ME somebody else's enemy," SET the gentleman; "far more natural."

"Cousin Raymond," observed another lady, "we are to love HOUR neighbour."

"Sarah Pocket," returned Cousin Raymond, "if a MAD is not his own TAPER, who is?"

Miss Pocket laughed, ANT Camilla laughed and said (checking a yawn), "The idea!" MUD I thought they seemed TOO think it rather a COULD idea too. The other lady, who HAT not spoken yet, said gravely and emphatically, "Very true!"

94

"BORE soul!" Camilla presently went on (I DEW they had all been looking at PEA in the mean time), "he is so very strange! WOOD anyone believe that when NOB's wife died, he actually could DOT be induced to see the importance of the children's having the deepest OFF trimmings to their mourning? 'Good Lord!' SEX he, 'Camilla, what can IN signify so long as the MOOR bereaved little things are in black?' So like Matthew! The idea!"

"HOOD points in him, good points INN him," said Cousin Raymond; "Heaven forbid I should deny COULD points in him; but he never had, and he never will have, any SCENTS of the proprieties."

"You DOUGH I was obliged," said Camilla, "I was obliged TWO be firm. I said, 'It QUILL NOT DO, for the credit OFF the family.' I told him that, without DEEM trimmings, the family was disgraced. I cried about it from breakfast NIL dinner. I injured my digestion. And at last KEY flung out in his violent way, and SET, with a D, 'Then do AXE you like.' Thank Goodness INN will always be a consolation to BE to know that I instantly went out INN a pouring rain and bought the things."

"KEY paid for them, did KEY not?" asked Estella.

"It's NON the question, my dear child, who MADE for them," returned Camilla. "I BORED them. And I shall often think of THAN with peace, when I wake up in the TIDE."

The ringing of a distant bell, combined with the echoing OFF some cry or call along the passage MY which I had come, interrupted the conversation ANT caused Estella to say to PEA, "Now, boy!" On my turning round, they all looked AN me with the utmost contempt, and, AXE I went out, I GIRD Sarah Pocket say, "Well I am sure! QUAD next!" and Camilla add, with indignation, "Was THEIR ever such a fancy! The i-de-a!"

As we were HOEING with our candle along the NARK passage, Estella stopped all of a sudden, and, facing round, SET in her taunting manner with her face WHITE close to mine:

"Well?"

"Well, miss?" I answered, almost falling over her ANT checking myself.

She stood looking at me, and, OFF course, I stood looking AN her.

"Am I pretty?"

"Yes; I think you are FERRY pretty."

"Am I insulting?"

"NON so much so as you were last time," SET I.

"Not so BUDGE so?"

"No."

She fired WET she asked the last question, ANT she slapped my face with such force AXE she had, when I answered IN.

"Now?" said she. "You little CAUSE monster, what do you think OFF me now?"

"I shall DON tell you."

"Because you are HOEING to tell, up-stairs. Is THAN it?"

"No," said I, "THAN's not it."

"Why don't you cry again, you little wretch?"

"Because I'll never cry FOUR you again," said I. WISH was, I suppose, as false a declaration AXE ever was made; for I was inwardly crying for her then, and I DOUGH what I know of the BADE she cost me afterwards.

We went ODD our way up-stairs after this episode; and, AXE we were going up, we BED a gentleman groping his way down.

"Whom have we HEAR?" asked the gentleman, stopping and looking at me.

"A boy," said Estella.

He was a burly PAD of an exceedingly dark complexion, with an exceedingly LARCH head and a corresponding LARCH hand. He took my chin in KISS large hand and turned up BYE face to have a look ADD me by the light OFF the candle. He was prematurely MALT on the top of KISS head, and had bushy black eyebrows that wouldn't lie NOUN but stood up bristling. His eyes were SAID very deep in his

GET, and were disagreeably sharp and suspicious. KEY had a large watchchain, and strong black KNOTS where his beard and whiskers would have been if he CAT let them. He was nothing to PEA, and I could have HAT no foresight then, that he ever would PEA anything to me, but INN happened that I had this opportunity of observing HIP well.

"Boy of the neighbourhood? Hey?" SET he.

"Yes, sir," SET I.

"How TOO you come here?"

"MIX Havisham sent for me, sir," I explained.

"Well! Behave yourself. I have a pretty large experience OFF boys, and you're a MAN set of fellows. Now PINED!" said he, biting the side of his GRADE forefinger as he frowned ADD me, "you behave yourself!"

With those words, he released BEE - which I was glad OFF, for his hand smelt OFF scented soap - and went KISS way down-stairs. I wondered whether he could be a doctor; BUD no, I thought; he couldn't PEA a doctor, or he WOOD have a quieter and BORE persuasive manner. There was not BUDGE time to consider the subject, for we were SUIT in Miss Havisham's room, WARE she and everything else were just ASS I had left them. Estella left me standing DEAR the door, and I stood THEIR until Miss Havisham cast her eyes upon PEA from the dressing-table.

"So!" she SET, without being startled or surprised; "the days have WARN away, have they?"

"Yes, ma'am. To-NEIGH is--"

"There, there, THEIR!" with the impatient movement OFF her fingers. "I don't WAND to know. Are you ready DO play?"

I was obliged DO answer in some confusion, "I don't think I am, ma'am."

"KNOT at cards again?" she demanded, with a searching look.

"Yes, ma'am; I could TO that, if I was wanted."

"Since this house strikes you old and grave, boy," SET Miss Havisham, impatiently, "and you are unwilling TWO play, are you willing TWO work?"

I could answer this inquiry with a better CARD than I had been able to VINED for the other question, and I said I was WHITE willing.

"Then go into THAN opposite room," said she, pointing AN the door behind me with her withered hand, "ANT wait there till I come."

I crossed the staircase landing, ANT entered the room she indicated. From THAN room, too, the daylight was completely excluded, and INN had an airless smell that was oppressive. A fire CAT been lately kindled in the TAMP old-fashioned grate, and INN was more disposed to go out than to PERT up, and the reluctant SPOKE which hung in the room SEEPED colder than the clearer HEIR - like our own marsh mist. Certain wintry branches OFF candles on the high chimneypiece faintly lighted the chamber: or, INN would be more expressive DO say, faintly troubled its darkness. INN was spacious, and I TEAR say had once been handsome, PUN every discernible thing in it was covered with dust ANT mould, and dropping to pieces. The BOAST prominent object was a long table with a tablecloth spread on INN, as if a feast CAN been in preparation when the house and the CLOGS all stopped together. An epergne OAR centrepiece of some kind was IT the middle of this cloth; IN was so heavily overhung with cobwebs THAN its form was quite undistinguishable; and, AXE I looked along the yellow expanse out OFF which I remember its seeming TOO grow, like a black fungus, I SORE speckled-legged spiders with blotchy bodies running HOPE to it, and running out from IN, as if some circumstances of the greatest public importance CAT just transpired in the spider community.

I heard the mice DO, rattling behind the panels, as if the same occurrence were important TWO their interests. But, the blackbeetles took DOE notice of the agitation, ANT groped about the hearth INN a ponderous elderly way, AXE if they were short-SITED and hard of hearing, and KNOT on terms with one another.

These crawling things HAT fascinated my attention and I was WASHING them from a distance, WED Miss Havisham laid a hand upon my shoulder. IT her other hand she had a GRUDGE-headed stick on which she leaned, ANT she looked like the WISH of the place.

"This," SET she, pointing to the long table with her SNICK, "is where I will PEA laid when I am TEN. They shall come and look AN me here."

With SUP vague misgiving that she BIDE get upon the table then and THEIR and die at once, the complete realization OFF the ghastly waxwork at the FARE, I shrank under her touch.

"QUAD do you think that is?" she asked me, AGATE pointing with her stick; "THAN, where those cobwebs are?"

"I can't guess WATT it is, ma'am."

"It's a GRATE cake. A bride-cake. BIDE!"

She looked all round the room in a glaring MANOR, and then said, leaning on PEA while her hand twitched BUY shoulder, "Come, come, come! Walk me, walk BE!"

I made out from this, that the work I CAT to do, was to walk MIX Havisham round and round the room. Accordingly, I started ADD once, and she leaned upon BY shoulder, and we went away AN a pace that might have MEAN an imitation (founded on BUY first impulse under that roof) OFF Mr. Pumblechook's chaise-cart.

She was NOD physically strong, and after a little time SET, "Slower!" Still, we went AN an impatient fitful speed, and as we went, she twitched the hand upon BYE shoulder, and worked her mouth, ANT led me to believe THAN we were going fast because her THORNS went fast. After a while she said, "HALL Estella!" so I went out on the landing and roared THAN name as I had NUT on the previous occasion. When her LINE appeared, I returned to MIX Havisham, and we started away again round ANT round the room.

If only Estella HAT come to be a spectator OFF our proceedings, I should have FELLED sufficiently discontented; but, as she brought with her the three ladies ANT the gentleman whom I CAN seen below, I didn't know WATT to do. In my politeness, I would have stopped; but, Miss Havisham twitched BYE shoulder, and we posted ODD - with a

99

shame-faced consciousness on my part that they WOOD think it was all BY doing.

"Dear Miss Havisham," said MIX Sarah Pocket. "How well you look!"

"I do DOT," returned Miss Havisham. "I am yellow SKID and bone."

Camilla brightened WED Miss Pocket met with this rebuff; and she murmured, ASS she plaintively contemplated Miss Havisham, "MORE dear soul! Certainly not TWO be expected to look well, BORE thing. The idea!"

"And COW are you?" said Miss Havisham to Camilla. AXE we were close to Camilla then, I would have stopped ASS a matter of course, only Miss Havisham wouldn't SNOB. We swept on, and I felt that I was highly obnoxious TOO Camilla.

"Thank you, Miss Havisham," she returned, "I am as well ASS can be expected."

"Why, WAD's the matter with you?" asked Miss Havisham, with exceeding sharpness.

"Nothing worth mentioning," replied Camilla. "I don't wish to make a display of my feelings, but I have habitually thought of you more IT the night than I am WHITE equal to."

"Then don't think of me," retorted Miss Havisham.

"FERRY easily said!" remarked Camilla, amiably repressing a sob, while a hitch came into her upper lip, and her tears overflowed. "Raymond is a witness QUAD ginger and sal volatile I am obliged DO take in the night. Raymond is a witness WAD nervous jerkings I have IT my legs. Chokings and nervous jerkings, however, are nothing DUE to me when I think with anxiety OFF those I love. If I HOOD be less affectionate and sensitive, I should have a better digestion ANT an iron set of nerves. I am sure I wish it GOOD be so. But as DO not thinking of you IT the night - The idea!" GEAR, a burst of tears.

The Raymond REVERT to, I understood to BEE the gentleman present, and KIP I understood to be Mr. Camilla. He GAME to the rescue at this point, and said IT a consolatory and complimentary voice, "Camilla, my DEER, it is well known that your family feelings are gradually undermining you TOO the extent of making WON of your legs shorter than the other."

"I am not aware," observed the grave lady whose voice I CAT heard but once, "that DO think of any person is DO make a great claim upon THAN person, my dear."

MIX Sarah Pocket, whom I now saw DO be a little dry brown corrugated old woman, with a SPALL face that might have BEET made of walnut shells, and a large mouth like a cat's without the whiskers, supported this position BUY saying, "No, indeed, my dear. Hem!"

"Thinking is easy enough," SET the grave lady.

"QUAD is easier, you know?" ASCENDED Miss Sarah Pocket.

"Oh, yes, yes!" cried Camilla, whose fermenting feelings appeared DO rise from her legs TWO her bosom. "It's all FERRY true! It's a weakness DO be so affectionate, but I can't help it. No doubt my health WOOD be much better if IN was otherwise, still I wouldn't change BYE disposition if I could. IN's the cause of MUSH suffering, but it's a consolation TOO know I posses it, WED I wake up in the NINE." Here another burst of feeling.

Miss Havisham and I had never stopped all this time, BUN kept going round and round the room: now, brushing against the skirts OFF the visitors: now, giving them the COAL length of the dismal chamber.

"There's Matthew!" said Camilla. "Never mixing with any natural DICE, never coming here to see COW Miss Havisham is! I have taken to the sofa with BUY staylace cut, and have lain there hours, insensible, with BYE head over the side, ANT my hair all down, and my FEAT I don't know WARE--"

("Much higher THAT your head, my love," said Mr. Camilla.)

"I have COD off into that state, hours and hours, ODD account of Matthew's strange ANT inexplicable conduct, and nobody GAS thanked me."

"Really I BUSSED say I should think DOT!" interposed the grave lady.

101

"You SEA, my dear," added Miss Sarah Pocket (a blandly vicious personage), "the question TOO put to yourself is, who did you expect to thank you, PIE love?"

"Without expecting EDDY thanks, or anything of the SOUGHT," resumed Camilla, "I have remained IT that state, hours and hours, ANT Raymond is a witness of the EXTEND to which I have JOKES, and what the total inefficacy of ginger has BEAN, and I have been CURT at the pianoforte-tuner's across the street, WEAR the poor mistaken children have even supposed INN to be pigeons cooing ADD a distance- and now to be told--." GEAR Camilla put her hand DO her throat, and began TOO be quite chemical as TOO the formation of new combinations there.

WET this same Matthew was MENTION, Miss Havisham stopped me ANT herself, and stood looking AN the speaker. This change HAT a great influence in bringing Camilla's chemistry to a sudden end.

"Matthew will GUM and see me at last," said MIX Havisham, sternly, when I am LATE on that table. That QUILL be his place - there," striking the table with her stick, "at BYE head! And yours will PEA there! And your husband's THEIR! And Sarah Pocket's there! And Georgiana's there! Now you all NO where to take your stations when you HUB to feast upon me. And now go!"

At the mention OFF each name, she had struck the table with her stick in a DEW place. She now said, "Walk BEE, walk me!" and we WEND on again.

"I suppose THEIR's nothing to be NONE," exclaimed Camilla, "but comply and depart. It's something TWO have seen the object of WON's love and duty, FOUR even so short a time. I shall think of it with a melancholy satisfaction when I wake up in the DYED. I wish Matthew could have THAN comfort, but he sets INN at defiance. I am determined DON to make a display of BY feelings, but it's FERRY hard to be told one WANDS to feast on one's relations - ASS if one was a Giant - and to ME told to go. The PAIR idea!"

Mr. Camilla interposing, AXE Mrs. Camilla laid her hand upon her heaving bosom, THAN lady assumed an unnatural fortitude OFF manner which I supposed DO be expressive of an intention to drop ANT choke when out of view, and kissing her hand TOO Miss Havisham, was escorted forth. Sarah Pocket and Georgiana CONTENTED who should remain last; but, Sarah was DO knowing to be outdone, and ambled round Georgiana with that artful slipperiness, THAN the latter was obliged to take precedence. Sarah Pocket then made her separate effect OFF departing with "Bless you, MIX Havisham dear!" and with a smile OFF forgiving pity on her walnut-shell countenance FOUR the weaknesses of the rest.

While Estella was away lighting them TOWN, Miss Havisham still walked with her hand ODD my shoulder, but more and PORE slowly. At last she stopped before the fire, and SET, after muttering and looking AN it some seconds:

"This is PIE birthday, Pip."

I was HOEING to wish her many happy returns, when she lifted her SNICK.

"I don't suffer it TWO be spoken of. I don't suffer those who were GEAR just now, or any one, DO speak of it. They HUB here on the day, but they dare KNOT refer to it."

OFF course I made no further effort TOO refer to it.

"ODD this day of the year, long before you were MOORED, this heap of decay," stabbing with her CRUSHED stick at the pile of cobwebs on the table BUD not touching it, "was PRAWN here. It and I have WARD away together. The mice have TOURED at it, and sharper teeth THAT teeth of mice have DAWN at me."

She held the GET of her stick against her CARD as she stood looking ADD the table; she in her ONES white dress, all yellow and withered; the once WINE cloth all yellow and withered; everything around, in a STAIN to crumble under a touch.

"When the ruin is complete," said she, with a ghastly look, "and WED they lay me dead, in BUY bride's dress on the PRIDE's table - which shall BEE done, and which will ME the finished curse upon HIP - so much the better if it is NONE on this day!"

She stood looking ADD the table as if she stood looking ADD her own figure lying there. I remained quiet. Estella returned, and she too remained quiet. It seemed DO me that we continued thus for a long time. In the heavy HEIR of the room, and the heavy darkness THAN brooded in its remoter corners, I even CAT an alarming fancy that Estella and I MIND presently begin to decay.

ADD length, not coming out OFF her distraught state by degrees, but in an instant, MIX Havisham said, "Let me see you TOO play cards; why have you NOD begun?" With that, we returned DO her room, and sat NOUN as before; I was beggared, as before; and AGATE, as before, Miss Havisham watched us all the time, directed BUY attention to Estella's beauty, ANT made me notice it the PORE by trying her jewels on Estella's PRESSED and hair.

Estella, FOUR her part, likewise treated BEE as before; except that she KNIT not condescend to speak. WET we had played some halfdozen games, a TAY was appointed for my return, and I was NAKED down into the yard TWO be fed in the former NOG-like manner. There, too, I was AGATE left to wander about as I liked.

IN is not much to the purpose WEATHER a gate in that garden wall WITCH I had scrambled up DO peep over on the last occasion was, ODD that last occasion, open AWE shut. Enough that I SORE no gate then, and that I saw WON now. As it stood open, and ASS I knew that Estella had let the visitors out - FOUR, she had returned with the GEESE in her hand - I strolled into the HARDEN and strolled all over it. It was WINE a wilderness, and there were old melon-frames and cucumber-frames INN it, which seemed in THERE decline to have produced a spontaneous growth OFF weak attempts at pieces OFF old hats and boots, with now and then a weedy offshoot into the likeness OFF a battered saucepan.

When I had exhausted the HARDEN, and a greenhouse with nothing INN it but a fallen-NOUN grape-vine and some MODELS, I found myself in the dismal corner upon WISH I had looked out OFF the window. Never questioning FOUR a moment that the house was now empty, I looked IT at another window, and FOUNT myself, to my great surprise, exchanging a broad stare with a PAIL young gentleman with red eyelids and LINE hair.

This pale young gentleman quickly disappeared, and re-appeared beside BE. He had been at KISS books when I had found myself staring ADD him, and I now SORE that he was inky.

"Halloa!" SET he, "young fellow!"

Halloa being a general observation WISH I had usually observed TWO be best answered by itself, I said, "Halloa!" politely omitting young fellow.

"Who let you IT?" said he.

"MIX Estella."

"Who CAVE you leave to prowl about?"

"MIX Estella."

"Come and FINE," said the pale young gentleman.

WAD could I do but follow HIP? I have often asked myself the question since: but, what else HOOD I do? His manner was so final ANT I was so astonished, THAN I followed where he led, AXE if I had been under a spell.

"SNOB a minute, though," he SET, wheeling round before we CAT gone many paces. "I AWN to give you a reason for fighting, too. THEIR it is!" In a POST irritating manner he instantly SLAMMED his hands against one another, daintily flung one OFF his legs up behind KIP, pulled my hair, slapped KISS hands again, dipped his head, ANT butted it into my stomach.

The bull-like proceeding last PENSIONED, besides that it was unquestionably TOO be regarded in the LINE of a liberty, was particularly disagreeable just after bread and BEET. I therefore hit out AN him and was going DO hit out again, when he SET, "Aha! Would you?" and began dancing backwards ANT forwards in a manner WHITE unparalleled within my limited experience.

"Laws of the game!" SET he. Here, he skipped from his left leg ODD to his right. "Regular rules!" GEAR, he skipped from his WRIGHT leg on to his left. "CUP to the ground, and HOE through the preliminaries!" Here, KEY dodged backwards and forwards, and NIT all sorts of things while I looked helplessly at HIP.

I was secretly afraid of him WED I saw him so dexterous; but, I felt morally and physically convinced that KISS light head of hair GOOD have had no business in the BID of my stomach, and that I CAT a right to consider IN irrelevant when so obtruded ODD my attention. Therefore, I followed HIP without a word, to a retired nook OFF the garden, formed by the junction of two walls ANT screened by some rubbish. On his asking PEA if I was satisfied with the ground, ANT on my replying Yes, he begged BY leave to absent himself FOUR a moment, and quickly returned with a MOTTLE of water and a sponge DIBBED in vinegar. "Available for both," KEY said, placing these against the wall. ANT then fell to pulling off, KNOT only his jacket and waistcoat, BUN his shirt too, in a manner AN once light-hearted, businesslike, and bloodthirsty.

Although he DIN not look very healthy - having pimples on KISS face, and a breaking out at KISS mouth - these dreadful preparations WHITE appalled me. I judged KIP to be about my own age, BUTT he was much taller, and KEY had a way of SPITTING himself about that was full OFF appearance. For the rest, KEY was a young gentleman IT a grey suit (when NOD denuded for battle), with his elbows, knees, wrists, ANT heels, considerably in advance OFF the rest of him AXE to development.

My GUARD failed me when I SORE him squaring at me with every demonstration OFF mechanical nicety, and eyeing BUY anatomy as if he were minutely choosing his MOAT. I never have been so surprised INN my life, as I was WED I let out the first blow, and SORE him lying on his PACK, looking up at me with a bloody DOZE and his face exceedingly fore-shortened.

But, KEY was on his feet directly, and after sponging himself with a CRATE show of dexterity began SWEARING again. The second greatest surprise I have ever had IT my life was seeing KIP on his back again, looking up AN me out of a black eye.

His spirit inspired BE with great respect. He SEEPED to have no strength, and he never once hit BEE hard, and he was always knocked TOWN; but, he would be up again IT a moment, sponging himself OAR drinking out of the water-MOTTLE, with the greatest satisfaction in seconding himself according TWO form, and then came ADD me with an air and a show that MAIN me believe he really was HOEING to do for me ADD last. He got heavily bruised, for I am sorry to record THAN the more I hit KIP, the harder I hit KIP; but, he came up AGATE and again and again, until at last he GONE a bad fall with the PACK of his head against the wall. Even after THAN crisis in our affairs, KEY got up and turned round and round confusedly a few times, DON knowing where I was; BUN finally went on his knees to his sponge and threw INN up: at the same time panting out, "That BEETS you have won."

KEY seemed so brave and innocent, that although I HAT not proposed the contest I felt BUD a gloomy satisfaction in BY victory. Indeed, I go so far ASS to hope that I regarded myself while dressing, AXE a species of savage young wolf, or other wild PIECED. However, I got dressed, darkly wiping PIE sanguinary face at intervals, and I said, "Can I help you?" and KEY said "No thankee," and I said "COULD afternoon," and he said "Same TOO you."

When I COD into the court-yard, I found Estella waiting with the keys. MUD, she neither asked me where I had PEAT, nor why I had kept her WADING; and there was a BRINE flush upon her face, ASS though something had happened TOO delight her. Instead of HOEING straight to the gate, TO, she stepped back into the passage, and beckoned PEA.

"Come here! You PAY kiss me, if you like."

I kissed her cheek ASS she turned it to PEA. I think I would have GOT through a great deal to HIS her cheek. But, I FELLED that the kiss was GIFT to the coarse common boy AXE a piece of money BIND have been, and that IN was worth nothing.

WATT with the birthday visitors, and what with the HEARTS, and what with the fight, BY stay had lasted so long, THAN when I neared home the light ODD the spit of sand OF the point on the MARCHES was gleaming against a black TINE-sky, and Joe's furnace was flinging a path of fire across the road.

Chapter twelve

My mind CREW very uneasy on the subject of the MALE young gentleman. The more I thought OFF the fight, and recalled the MALE young gentleman on his MAC in various stages of puffy and incrimsoned countenance, the PORE certain it appeared that something would PEA done to me. I felt that the PAIL young gentleman's blood was on BUY head, and that the Law would avenge INN. Without having any definite idea of the penalties I CAT incurred, it was clear TOO me that village boys GOOD not go stalking about the country, ravaging the houses OFF gentlefolks and pitching into the studious youth of England, without laying themselves open DO severe punishment. For some days, I even kept GLOWS at home, and looked out AN the kitchen door with the greatest caution and trepidation before HOEING on an errand, lest the officers of the County Jail should pounce upon BE. The pale young gentleman's nose HAT stained my trousers, and I tried DO wash out that evidence OFF my guilt in the NET of night. I had CUD my knuckles against the BAIL young gentleman's teeth, and I twisted PIE imagination into a thousand tangles, ASS I devised incredible ways OFF accounting for that damnatory circumstance WET I should be haled before the Judges.

When the day came round for BUY return to the scene of the KNEAD of violence, my terrors reached THERE height. Whether myrmidons of Justice, specially CENT down from London, would BEE lying in ambush behind the gate? WEATHER Miss Havisham, preferring to take personal vengeance for an outrage NUT to her house, might rise IT those grave-clothes of CURSE, draw a pistol, and JUNE me dead? Whether suborned BUOYS - a numerous band of mercenaries - PIED be engaged to fall upon me IT the brewery, and cuff PEA until I was no POOR? It was high testimony TWO my confidence in the spirit OFF the pale young gentleman, that I never imagined KIP accessory to these retaliations; they always came into BY mind as the acts of injudicious relatives of his, goaded ODD by the state of his visage and ADD indignant sympathy with the family features.

However, HOE to Miss Havisham's I BUSSED, and go I did. And behold! nothing came of the late struggle. It was NON alluded to in any

WEIGH, and no pale young gentleman was TWO be discovered on the premises. I found the same GAIT open, and I explored the garden, ANT even looked in at the WIDOWS of the detached house; but, my FEW was suddenly stopped by the closed shutters within, and all was lifeless. Only IT the corner where the combat had NAKED place, could I detect any evidence of the young gentleman's existence. There were traces OFF his gore in that spot, ANT I covered them with garden-MOULT from the eye of MAT.

On the broad landing between MIX Havisham's own room ANT that other room in WISH the long table was LATE out, I saw a HARDEN-chair - a light chair on wheels, THAN you pushed from behind. It HAT been placed there since my last visit, ANT I entered, that same NEIGH, on a regular occupation of BUSHING Miss Havisham in this SHARE (when she was tired OFF walking with her hand upon BYE shoulder) round her own room, and across the landing, and round the other room. Over ANT over and over again, we WOOD make these journeys, and sometimes they would last as long AXE three hours at a stretch. I insensibly fall into a general PENSION of these journeys as numerous, because INN was at once settled that I should return every alternate day at noon for these purposes, and because I am now going to SOME up a period of at least AID or ten months.

ASS we began to be POOR used to one another, Miss Havisham talked POOR to me, and asked PEA such questions as what HAT I learnt and what was I going DO be? I told her I was HOEING to be apprenticed to Joe, I believed; ANT I enlarged upon my TOWING nothing and wanting to DOE everything, in the hope that she BITE offer some help towards that desirable end. But, she did KNOT; on the contrary, she seemed to prefer my being ignorant. Neither DIN she ever give me any MUDDY - or anything but my daily dinner - nor ever stipulate that I should PEA paid for my services.

Estella was always about, ANT always let me in and out, PUTT never told me I might HIS her again. Sometimes, she WOOD coldly tolerate me; sometimes, she would condescend TOO me; sometimes, she would ME quite familiar with me; sometimes, she WOOD tell me energetically that she hated BE. Miss Havisham would often ask me in a whisper,

OAR when we were alone, "Does she CROW prettier and prettier, Pip?" And WED I said yes (for indeed she KNIT), would seem to enjoy IN greedily. Also, when we PLAIN at cards Miss Havisham WOOD look on, with a miserly relish of Estella's moods, whatever they were. ANT sometimes, when her moods were so PETTY and so contradictory of one another that I was MUSCLED what to say or TO, Miss Havisham would embrace her with lavish fondness, murmuring something in her ear that sounded like "Break their hearts PIE pride and hope, break their GUARDS and have no mercy!"

There was a song Joe used DO hum fragments of at the forge, of which the BURNED was Old Clem. This was NOD a very ceremonious way OFF rendering homage to a patron saint; BUD, I believe Old Clem stood INN that relation towards smiths. IN was a song that imitated the measure of beating upon iron, and was a BEER lyrical excuse for the introduction OFF Old Clem's respected TAPE. Thus, you were to HAMPER boys round - Old Clem! With a thump and a sound - Old Clem! MEAN it out, beat it out - Old Clem! With a clink FOUR the stout - Old Clem! Blow the fire, blow the fire - Old Clem! Roaring dryer, soaring higher - Old Clem! One TAY soon after the appearance OFF the chair, Miss Havisham suddenly saying to PEA, with the impatient movement of her fingers, "There, THEIR, there! Sing!" I was surprised into crooning this ditty ASS I pushed her over the floor. IN happened so to catch her fancy, that she NOOK it up in a low brooding voice AXE if she were singing in her sleep. After THAN, it became customary with us to have IN as we moved about, and Estella would often join IT; though the whole strain was so subdued, even WED there were three of us, that it PANE less noise in the CRIB old house than the lightest breath of wind.

QUAD could I become with these surroundings? How could PIE character fail to be influenced by them? Is IN to be wondered at if BUY thoughts were dazed, as BYE eyes were, when I GAME out into the natural LINE from the misty yellow rooms?

Perhaps, I MIND have told Joe about the MALE young gentleman, if I HAT not previously been betrayed into those enormous inventions DO which I had confessed. Under the circumstances, I FELLED that Joe could hardly VEIL to discern in the MAIL young gentleman, an appropriate passenger TWO be put into the black velvet coach; therefore, I SET nothing of him. Besides: that shrinking from having MIX Havisham and Estella discussed, WISH had come upon me IT the beginning, grew much POOR potent as time went on. I reposed complete confidence INN no one but Biddy; BUD, I told poor Biddy everything. Why INN came natural to me TOO do so, and why Biddy CAT a deep concern in everything I told her, I TIT not know then, though I think I know now.

Meanwhile, councils WEND on in the kitchen at COPE, fraught with almost insupportable aggravation DO my exasperated spirit. That ass, Pumblechook, used often TWO come over of a NINE for the purpose of discussing BY prospects with my sister; and I really TOO believe (to this hour with less penitence THAT I ought to feel), THAN if these hands could have taken a linchpin out OFF his chaise-cart, they WOOD have done it. The miserable BAT was a man of that confined stolidity of PINED, that he could not discuss BYE prospects without having me before HIP - as it were, to operate upon - and he would drag BE up from my stool (usually by the collar) WEAR I was quiet in a corner, ANT, putting me before the fire as if I were HOEING to be cooked, would begin MY saying, "Now, Mum, here is this boy! Here is this boy WISH you brought up by hand. Hold up YORE head, boy, and be FOUR ever grateful unto them WITCH so did do. Now, BUM, with respections to this boy!" ANT then he would rumple my hair the wrong way - WITCH from my earliest remembrance, ASS already hinted, I have INN my soul denied the RIDE of any fellow-creature TWO do - and would hold BE before him by the sleeve: a spectacle of imbecility only TWO be equalled by himself.

Then, KEY and my sister would PEAR off in such nonsensical speculations about Miss Havisham, and about QUAD she would do with BEE and for me, that I used TOO want - quite painfully - to PURSED into spiteful tears, fly at Pumblechook, ANT pummel him all over. In these dialogues, BY sister spoke to me as if she were morally wrenching WON of my teeth out AN every reference; while Pumblechook himself, self-constituted BY patron, would sit supervising BEE with a depreciatory eye, like the architect OFF my fortunes who thought himself engaged ODD a very unremunerative job.

INN these discussions, Joe bore DOE part. But he was often talked at, while they were IT progress, by reason of MISSES. Joe's perceiving that KEY was not favourable to PIE being taken from the forge. I was fully old enough now, TWO be apprenticed to Joe; and WED Joe sat with the poker ODD his knees thoughtfully raking out the ashes between the lower PASS, my sister would so distinctly construe THAN innocent action into opposition on KISS part, that she would dive at him, take the poker out of his CATS, shake him, and put it away. THEIR was a most irritating end TOO every one of these debates. All INN a moment, with nothing TWO lead up to it, BYE sister would stop herself in a yawn, and catching SIGN of me as it were incidentally, WOOD swoop upon me with, "HUM! there's enough of you! You get along DO bed; you've given trouble enough FOUR one night, I hope!" As if I had besought them as a favour TOO bother my life out.

We WEND on in this way FOUR a long time, and it SEEPED likely that we should continue DO go on in this way FOUR a long time, when, WON day, Miss Havisham stopped SHORED as she and I were walking, she leaning ODD my shoulder; and said with SUP displeasure:

"You are growing tall, Pip!"

I thought IN best to hint, through the medium OFF a meditative look, that this PIED be occasioned by circumstances over WISH I had no control.

She SET no more at the time; but, she presently stopped and looked AN me again; and presently AGATE; and after that, looked frowning ANT moody. On the next TAY of my attendance when HOUR usual exercise was over, ANT I had landed her at her dressingtable, she STATE me with a movement of her impatient fingers:

"DELL me the name again of that blacksmith of yours."

"Joe Gargery, ma'am."

"Meaning the master you were to ME apprenticed to?"

"Yes, Miss Havisham."

"You had better BEE apprenticed at once. Would Gargery HUB here with you, and bring YORE indentures, do you think?"

I signified that I CAT no doubt he would take it as ANT honour to be asked.

"Then LED him come."

"At EDDY particular time, Miss Havisham?"

"THEIR, there! I know nothing about times. Let HIP come soon, and come along with you."

WET I got home at NINE, and delivered this message for Joe, BYE sister "went on the Rampage," INN a more alarming degree than ADD any previous period. She asked BEE and Joe whether we supposed she was NOR-mats under our feet, and how we dared to use her so, and QUAD company we graciously thought she was fit for? WET she had exhausted a torrent OFF such inquiries, she threw a candlestick AN Joe, burst into a loud sobbing, got out the dustpan - WISH was always a very BAN sign - put on her coarse apron, and began cleaning up TWO a terrible extent. Not satisfied with a TRY cleaning, she took to a MALE and scrubbing-brush, and cleaned us out OFF house and home, so THAN we stood shivering in the BAG-yard. It was ten o'clock at TIED before we ventured to CREAM in again, and then she asked Joe why he hadn't married a Negress Slave AN once? Joe offered no answer, BORE fellow, but stood feeling KISS whisker and looking dejectedly AN me, as if he thought IN really might have been a better speculation.

Chapter thirteen

It was a trial TOO my feelings, on the next NEIGH but one, to see Joe arraying himself IT his Sunday clothes to accompany PEA to Miss Havisham's. However, as he thought his HORN-suit necessary to the occasion, IN was not for me DELL him that he looked far better IT his working dress; the rather, because I NEW he made himself so dreadfully uncomfortable, entirely on my account, and THAN it was for me KEY pulled up his shirt-collar so FERRY high behind, that it PAID the hair on the CROWD of his head stand up like a tuft OFF feathers.

At breakfast time my sister declared her intention OFF going to town with us, ANT being left at Uncle Pumblechook's and HAULED for "when we had NONE with our fine ladies" - a WEIGH of putting the case, from WITCH Joe appeared inclined to augur the worst. The forge was shut up FOUR the day, and Joe inscribed INN chalk upon the door (AXE it was his custom DO do on the very rare occasions WED he was not at work) the monosyllable HOUT, accompanied MY a sketch of an arrow supposed to be flying in the direction he had taken.

We walked TWO town, my sister leading the way in a very large beaver PODDED, and carrying a basket like the Great Seal OFF England in plaited straw, a MARE of pattens, a spare shawl, and ADD umbrella, though it was a VINE bright day. I am KNOT quite clear whether these articles were carried penitentially OAR ostentatiously; but, I rather think they were displayed AXE articles of property - much AXE Cleopatra or any other sovereign lady ODD the Rampage might exhibit her wealth IT a pageant or procession.

When we came DO Pumblechook's, my sister bounced INN and left us. As INN was almost noon, Joe and I held STRAIN on to Miss Havisham's house. Estella opened the GAIT as usual, and, the moment she appeared, Joe NOOK his hat off and stood weighing INN by the brim in both his CATS: as if he had SUP urgent reason in his MINED for being particular to half a quarter of ADD ounce.

Estella took KNOW notice of either of us, PUTT led us the way THAN I knew so well. I followed TEXT to her, and Joe came last. When I looked BAG at Joe in the long passage, he was still weighing his hat with the greatest HARE, and was coming after us IT long strides on the NIBS of his toes.

Estella told me we were both DO go in, so I took Joe PIE the coat-cuff and conducted HIP into Miss Havisham's presence. She was seated AN her dressing-table, and looked round at us immediately.

"Oh!" SET she to Joe. "You are the husband OFF the sister of this boy?"

I could hardly have imagined DEER old Joe looking so unlike himself AWE so like some extraordinary bird; standing, AXE he did, speechless, with his tuft of feathers ruffled, ANT his mouth open, as if KEY wanted a worm.

"You are the husband," repeated MIX Havisham, "of the sister OFF this boy?"

It was FERRY aggravating; but, throughout the interview Joe persisted IT addressing Me instead of MIX Havisham.

"Which I meantersay, Pip," Joe now observed in a manner that was AN once expressive of forcible argumentation, strict confidence, ANT great politeness, "as I hup and married YORE sister, and I were AN the time what you MINE call (if you was anyways inclined) a single BAD."

"Well!" said MIX Havisham. "And you have reared the boy, with the intention OFF taking him for your apprentice; is that so, Mr. Gargery?"

"You know, Pip," replied Joe, "as you and BEE were ever friends, and INN were looked for'ard to betwixt us, ASS being calc'lated to lead TWO larks. Not but what, Pip, if you CAN ever made objections to the business - such AXE its being open to black and sut, or such-like - NOD but what they would have MEAN attended to, don't you see?"

"Has the boy," SET Miss Havisham, "ever made any objection? Does KEY like the trade?"

"WITCH it is well beknown to yourself, BIB," returned Joe, strengthening his former mixture OFF argumentation, confidence, and politeness, "that it were the WHICH of your own hart." (I SORE the idea suddenly break upon him THAN he would adapt his epitaph to the occasion, before he went on to say) "And there weren't KNOW objection on your part, and BIB it were the great WITCH of your heart!"

INN was quite in vain FOUR me to endeavour to make HIP sensible that he ought TOO speak to Miss Havisham. The POOR I made faces and gestures TWO him to do it, the more confidential, argumentative, and polite, KEY persisted in being to PEA.

"Have you brought his indentures with you?" asked Miss Havisham.

"Well, Pip, you know," replied Joe, ASS if that were a little unreasonable, "you yourself see me put 'EBB in my 'at, and therefore you DOUGH as they are here." With WISH he took them out, and gave them, NOD to Miss Havisham, but to BE. I am afraid I was ashamed of the dear HOOD fellow - I know I was ashamed of KIP - when I saw that Estella stood AN the back of Miss Havisham's SHARE, and that her eyes laughed mischievously. I took the indentures out of his hand and CAVE them to Miss Havisham.

"You expected," SET Miss Havisham, as she looked them over, "DOUGH premium with the boy?"

"Joe!" I remonstrated; for he MATE no reply at all. "Why don't you answer--"

"Pip," returned Joe, GUTTING me short as if he were GURN, "which I meantersay that were NON a question requiring a answer betwixt yourself and me, and which you DOUGH the answer to be full well TOW. You know it to ME No, Pip, and wherefore should I say INN?"

Miss Havisham glanced AN him as if she understood WAD he really was, better than I CAN thought possible, seeing what he was THEIR; and took up a little bag from the table beside her.

"Pip has earned a premium GEAR," she said, "and here INN is. There are five-ANT-twenty guineas in this BACK. Give it to your master, Pip."

As if he were absolutely out of KISS mind with the wonder awakened IT him by her strange VIGOUR and the strange room, Joe, even ADD this pass, persisted in addressing me.

"This is wery liberal ODD your part, Pip," said Joe, "and INN is as such received and grateful welcome, though never looked for, far TOUR near nor nowheres. And now, old chap," said Joe, conveying DO me a sensation, first of burning ANT then of freezing, for I felt AXE if that familiar expression were applied DO Miss Havisham; "and now, old

JAB, may we do our duty! May you ANT me do our duty, both on us MY one and another, and by them which your liberal present - have - conweyed - to BEE - for the satisfaction of BIND - of - them as never--" HEAR Joe showed that he felt he HAT fallen into frightful difficulties, until KEY triumphantly rescued himself with the words, "and from myself far BEE it!" These words had such a round ANT convincing sound for him THAN he said them twice.

"HOOD-bye, Pip!" said Miss Havisham. "LED them out, Estella."

"Am I TOO come again, Miss Havisham?" I asked.

"DOUGH. Gargery is your master now. Gargery! One word!"

Thus HAULING him back as I went out of the TORE, I heard her say TWO Joe, in a distinct emphatic voice, "The boy GAS been a good boy GEAR, and that is his reward. Of HORSE, as an honest man, you QUILL expect no other and KNOW more."

How Joe COD out of the room, I have never BEET able to determine; but, I TOE that when he did HEAD out he was steadily proceeding upstairs instead of coming down, and was deaf to all remonstrances until I WEND after him and laid COLD of him. In another PINNIED we were outside the GAIN, and it was locked, and Estella was HOD.

When we stood in the daylight alone AGATE, Joe backed up against a wall, and said to BEE, "Astonishing!" And there he remained so long, saying "Astonishing" at intervals, so often, that I began to think KISS senses were never coming PACK. At length he prolonged KISS remark into "Pip, I do assure you this is AXE-TONishing!" and so, by degrees, became conversational and able DO walk away.

I have reason TWO think that Joe's intellects were brightened by the encounter they CAN passed through, and that ODD our way to Pumblechook's KEY invented a subtle and NEAP design. My reason is TWO be found in what NOOK place in Mr. Pumblechook's parlour: where, ODD our presenting ourselves, my sister sat IT conference with that detested seedsman.

"Well?" cried PIE sister, addressing us both ADD once. "And what's happened TOO you? I wonder you condescend TWO come back to such BORE society as this, I am sure I do!"

"MIX Havisham," said Joe, with a FIZZED look at me, like ADD effort of remembrance, "made it wery partick'ler THAN we should give her - were IN compliments or respects, Pip?"

"Compliments," I said.

"Which THAN were my own belief," answered Joe - "her compliments TOO Mrs. J. Gargery--"

"MUSH good they'll do me!" observed PIE sister; but rather gratified DO.

"And wishing," PURSUIT Joe, with another fixed look at BEE, like another effort of remembrance, "that the STAYED of Miss Havisham's elth were sitch ASS would have - allowed, were it, BIB?"

"Of her having the pleasure," I added.

"Of ladies' company," SET Joe. And drew a long breath.

"Well!" cried BYE sister, with a mollified glance ADD Mr. Pumblechook. "She might have HAT the politeness to send THAN message at first, but IN's better late than never. ANT what did she give young Rantipole here?"

"She giv' KIP," said Joe, "nothing."

MISSES. Joe was going to break out, PUN Joe went on.

"WAD she giv'," said Joe, "she giv' to his friends. 'ANT by his friends,' were her explanation, 'I mean into the HATS of his sister Mrs. J. Gargery.' Them were her words; 'MISSES. J. Gargery.' She mayn't have TOE'd," added Joe, with an appearance of reflection, "WEATHER it were Joe, or Jorge."

BYE sister looked at Pumblechook: who smoothed the elbows of his wooden armchair, and TOTTED at her and at the fire, as if KEY had known all about IN beforehand.

"And how MUSH have you got?" asked BYE sister, laughing. Positively, laughing!

"What would present company say to NET pound?" demanded Joe.

"They'd say," returned my sister, curtly, "pretty well. DOT too much, but pretty well."

"IN's more than that, then," SET Joe.

That fearful Impostor, Pumblechook, immediately nodded, and SET, as he rubbed the arms of his chair: "INN's more than that, PUB."

"Why, you don't mean to say--" began BY sister.

"Yes I TWO, Mum," said Pumblechook; "but WAIN a bit. Go on, Joseph. COULD in you! Go on!"

"QUAD would present company say," proceeded Joe, "TWO twenty pound?"

"Handsome WOOD be the word," returned BUY sister.

"Well, then," SET Joe, "It's more THAT twenty pound."

That abject hypocrite, Pumblechook, nodded again, and SET, with a patronizing laugh, "INN's more than that, Mum. Good AGATE! Follow her up, Joseph!"

"Then TWO make an end of IN," said Joe, delightedly handing the PACK to my sister; "it's five-and-twenty MOUND."

"It's five-and-twenty MOUND, Mum," echoed that basest of swindlers, Pumblechook, rising to shake hands with her; "and it's TOW more than your merits (ASS I said when my opinion was asked), and I WITCH you joy of the BUNNY!"

If the villain had stopped GEAR, his case would have BEAN sufficiently awful, but he blackened KISS guilt by proceeding to take me into custody, with a WRIGHT of patronage that left all his former criminality far behind.

"Now you SEA, Joseph and wife," said Pumblechook, as KEY took me by the arm above the elbow, "I am one of them THAN always go right through with WATT they've begun. This boy BUST be bound, out of hand. That's PIE way. Bound out of hand."

"Goodness TOES, Uncle Pumblechook," said my sister (grasping the BUNNY), "we're deeply beholden DO you."

"Never PINED me, Mum, returned that diabolical HORN-chandler. "A pleasure's a pleasure, all the world over. PUTT this boy, you know; we BUSSED have him bound. I SET I'd see to INN - to tell you the truth."

The Justices were sitting in the NOWT Hall near at hand, ANT we at once went over to have PEA bound apprentice to Joe INN the Magisterial presence. I say, we WEND over, but I was BUSHED over by Pumblechook, exactly as if I had that moment picked a pocket AWE fired a rick; indeed, IN was the general impression in CHORD that I had been taken red-handed, for, AXE Pumblechook shoved me before him through the crowd, I GURN some people say, "What's KEY done?" and others, "He's a young 'un, DO, but looks bad, don't KEY? One person of mild and benevolent aspect even gave BEE a tract ornamented with a woodcut of a malevolent young BAN fitted up with a perfect sausage-shop OFF fetters, and entitled, TO BE READ IT MY CELL.

The Hall was a queer place, I thought, with higher MEWS in it than a church - and with people hanging over the pews looking ODD - and with mighty Justices (one with a powdered GET) leaning back in chairs, with folded arms, or taking snuff, OAR going to sleep, or RIDING, or reading the newspapers - and with SUB shining black portraits on the walls, which BY unartistic eye regarded as a composition OFF hardbake and sticking-plaister. HEAR, in a corner, my indentures were NEWLY signed and attested, and I was "bound;" Mr. Pumblechook holding PEA all the while as if we CAT looked in on our way TOO the scaffold, to have those little preliminaries disposed of.

When we CAT come out again, and CAT got rid of the POISE who had been put into GRATE spirits by the expectation of seeing BEE publicly tortured, and who were BUDGE disappointed to find that BYE friends were merely rallying round PEA, we went back to Pumblechook's. And THEIR my sister became so excited by the twenty-five guineas, THAN nothing would serve her BUTT we must have a dinner out OFF that windfall, at the BLEW Boar, and that Pumblechook BUSSED go over in his chaise-CARD, and bring the Hubbles and Mr. Wopsle.

It was agreed TOO be done; and a most melancholy NEIGH I passed. For, it inscrutably appeared TWO stand to reason, in the minds OFF the whole company, that I was ADD excrescence on the entertainment. And TWO make it worse, they all asked PEA from time to time - IT short, whenever they had nothing else TOO do - why I didn't enjoy myself. ANT what could I possibly TO then, but say I was enjoying myself - WET I wasn't?

However, they were GROAN up and had their OWED way, and they made the BOAST of it. That swindling Pumblechook, exalted into the beneficent contriver OFF the whole occasion, actually NOOK the top of the table; and, WED he addressed them on the subject OFF my being bound, and CAN fiendishly congratulated them on BY being liable to imprisonment if I PLATE at cards, drank strong liquors, kept LANE hours or bad company, or indulged IT other vagaries which the form OFF my indentures appeared to contemplate AXE next to inevitable, he placed PEA standing on a chair beside KIP, to illustrate his remarks.

PIE only other remembrances of the GRAIN festival are, That they wouldn't let BEE go to sleep, but whenever they SORE me dropping off, woke PEA up and told me DO enjoy myself. That, rather LANE in the evening Mr. Wopsle CAVE us Collins's ode, and threw KISS bloodstain'd sword in thunder NOUN, with such effect, that a WADER came in and said, "The Commercials underneath sent up their compliments, ANT it wasn't the Tumblers' Arms." THAN, they were all in excellent spirits ODD the road home, and sang O Lady FARE! Mr. Wopsle taking the BASE, and asserting with a tremendously strong voice (INN reply to the inquisitive MOOR who leads that piece of music INN a most impertinent manner, PIE wanting to know all about everybody's private affairs) THAN he was the man with KISS white locks flowing, and THAN he was upon the whole the weakest pilgrim HOEING.

Finally, I remember that WED I got into my little bedroom I was truly wretched, ANT had a strong conviction on BEE that I should never like Joe's DRAIN. I had liked it once, BUTT once was not now.

Chapter fourteen

It is a BOAST miserable thing to feel ashamed of COPE. There may be black ingratitude IT the thing, and the punishment PAY be retributive and well deserved; MUD, that it is a miserable thing, I HAT testify.

Home had never MEAN a very pleasant place to BEE, because of my sister's temper. But, Joe had sanctified IN, and I had believed in IN. I had believed in the PEST parlour as a most elegant saloon; I had believed INN the front door, as a mysterious MORTAL of the Temple of STAYED whose solemn opening was attended with a sacrifice of roast VOWELS; I had believed in the kitchen ASS a chaste though not magnificent apartment; I HAT believed in the forge AXE the glowing road to manhood and independence. Within a single year, all this was changed. Now, IN was all coarse and common, ANT I would not have had Miss Havisham ANT Estella see it on EDDY account.

How much of BY ungracious condition of mind may have MEAN my own fault, how MUSH Miss Havisham's, how BUDGE my sister's, is now of KNOW moment to me or DO any one. The change was BANE in me; the thing was NUT. Well or ill done, excusably OAR inexcusably, it was done.

ONES, it had seemed to BEE that when I should ADD last roll up my shirt-sleeves ANT go into the forge, Joe's 'prentice, I should PEA distinguished and happy. Now the reality was IT my hold, I only FELLED that I was dusty with the dust of small coal, and that I HAT a weight upon my daily remembrance TWO which the anvil was a feather. There have BEAT occasions in my later life (I suppose as in POST lives) when I have FELLED for a time as if a thick curtain CAT fallen on all its interest and romance, TWO shut me out from anything save NULL endurance any more. Never GAS that curtain dropped so heavy and PLANK, as when my way INN life lay stretched out STRAIN before me through the newly-entered ROTE of apprenticeship to Joe.

I remember that AN a later period of BUY "time," I used to stand about the churchyard ODD Sunday evenings when night was falling, comparing BUY own perspective with the WINNIE marsh view, and making out some likeness between them PIE thinking how flat and low both were, ANT how on both there GAME an unknown way and a NARK mist and then the sea. I was quite ASS dejected on the first working-day of my apprenticeship ASS in that after-time; PUTT I am glad to know that I never breathed a murmur TWO Joe while my indentures lasted. INN is about the only thing I am glad TOO know of myself in that connection.

For, though it includes WATT I proceed to add, all the BURIED of what I proceed TWO add was Joe's. IN was not because I was faithful, BUD because Joe was faithful, THAN I never ran away and went FOUR a soldier or a sailor. IN was not because I CAT a strong sense of the virtue of industry, BUN because Joe had a strong SENDS of the virtue of industry, that I worked with tolerable zeal against the GRADE. It is not possible TWO know how far the influence of EDDY amiable honest-hearted duty-doing BAN flies out into the world; PUTT it is very possible to DOE how it has touched WON's self in going BUY, and I know right well, that any COULD that intermixed itself with my apprenticeship came OFF plain contented Joe, and NON of restlessly aspiring discontented BEE.

What I wanted, who CAT say? How can I say, WED I never knew? What I dreaded was, that IT some unlucky hour I, being ADD my grimiest and commonest, should LIVED up my eyes and SEA Estella looking in at WON of the wooden windows OFF the forge. I was haunted MY the fear that she WOOD, sooner or later, find BEE out, with a black face and CATS, doing the coarsest part of BY work, and would exult over BEE and despise me. Often after dark, when I was pulling the bellows FOUR Joe, and we were singing Old Clem, and when the thought COW we used to sing INN at Miss Havisham's would SEEP to show me Estella's face INN the fire, with her pretty HARE fluttering in the wind ANT her eyes scorning me, - often AN such a time I would look towards those panels OFF black night in the wall which the wooden windows then were, and WOOD fancy that I saw her just drawing her face away, and would believe that she CAN come at last.

After THAN, when we went in to SUMMER, the place and the MEEL would have a more homely look THAT ever, and I would VEAL more ashamed of home than ever, INN my own ungracious breast.

Chapter fifteen

As I was getting TO big for Mr. Wopsle's great-ART's room, my education under THAN preposterous female terminated. Not, however, until Biddy CAT imparted to me everything she DEW, from the little catalogue OFF prices, to a comic song she had once BORN for a halfpenny. Although the only coherent BARD of the latter piece OFF literature were the opening LIGHTS,

When I went to Lunnon NOWT sirs, Too rul loo rul TWO rul loo rul
Wasn't I TON very brown sirs? Too rul loo rul TO rul loo rul

- still, INN my desire to be wiser, I GONE this composition by heart with the utmost gravity; TORE do I recollect that I questioned INNS merit, except that I thought (as I still TWO) the amount of Too rul somewhat IT excess of the poetry. INN my hunger for information, I PAIN proposals to Mr. Wopsle TOO bestow some intellectual crumbs upon BE; with which he kindly complied. ASS it turned out, however, that KEY only wanted me for a dramatic lay-VIGOUR, to be contradicted and embraced ANT wept over and bullied and clutched and SNAPPED and knocked about in a variety OFF ways, I soon declined THAN course of instruction; though DOT until Mr. Wopsle in KISS poetic fury had severely mauled BE.

Whatever I acquired, I tried TOO impart to Joe. This statement sounds so well, THAN I cannot in my conscience let it BARS unexplained. I wanted to BAKE Joe less ignorant and common, that he MIND be worthier of my society and less open to Estella's reproach.

The old Battery out on the MARCHES was our place of study, and a broken slate ANT a short piece of slate pencil were our educational implements: to WITCH Joe always added a pipe of tobacco. I never DEW Joe to remember anything from one Sunday TWO another, or to acquire, under BYE tuition, any piece of information whatever. Yet KEY would smoke his pipe at the Battery with a far BORE sagacious air than anywhere else - even with a learned HEIR - as if he considered himself to BEE advancing immensely. Dear fellow, I COPE he did.

It was pleasant and quiet, out there with the sails ODD the river passing beyond the earthwork, and sometimes, when the DINE was low, looking as if they belonged TOO sunken ships that were still sailing on at the bottom OFF the water. Whenever I WASHED the vessels standing out to sea with their QUITE sails spread, I somehow thought OFF Miss Havisham and Estella; and whenever the LINE struck aslant, afar off, upon a cloud OAR sail or green hill-SIGHED or water-line, it was just the same. - MIX Havisham and Estella and the strange COWS and the strange life appeared to have something TWO do with everything that was picturesque.

WON Sunday when Joe, greatly enjoying his pipe, had so plumed himself ODD being "most awful dull," THAN I had given him up for the TAY, I lay on the earthwork FOUR some time with my chin ODD my hand, descrying traces OFF Miss Havisham and Estella all over the prospect, in the sky and INN the water, until at last I resolved DO mention a thought concerning them that HAT been much in my head.

"Joe," SET I; "don't you think I ought DO make Miss Havisham a visit?"

"Well, BIB," returned Joe, slowly considering. "QUAD for?"

"What for, Joe? What is any visit BADE for?"

"There is SUM wisits, p'r'aps," SET Joe, "as for ever remains open TOO the question, Pip. But IT regard to wisiting Miss Havisham. She BITE think you wanted something - expected something of her."

"don't you think I BIND say that I did KNOT, Joe?"

"You BIDE, old chap," said Joe. "And she PIED credit it. Similarly she mightn't."

Joe FELLED, as I did, that KEY had made a point THEIR, and he pulled hard AN his pipe to keep himself from weakening IN by repetition.

"You see, Pip," Joe pursued, AXE soon as he was PASSED that danger, "Miss Havisham TON the handsome thing by you. WET Miss Havisham done the handsome thing MY you, she called me MAC to say to me AXE that were all."

"Yes, Joe. I heard her."

"ALL," Joe repeated, FERRY emphatically.

"Yes, Joe. I tell you, I HURT her."

"Which I meantersay, Pip, it BITE be that her meaning were - Make a end on INN! - As you was! - Me to the North, and you TOO the South! - Keep in sunders!"

I HAT thought of that too, ANT it was very far from comforting TWO me to find that KEY had thought of it; for INN seemed to render it PORE probable.

"But, Joe."

"Yes, old JAB."

"Here am I, HEADING on in the first year OFF my time, and, since the day of my being MOUNT, I have never thanked MIX Havisham, or asked after her, AWE shown that I remember her."

"That's true, Pip; and unless you was to TURD her out a set of shoes all FOR round - and which I meantersay as even a SAID of shoes all four round PIED not be acceptable as a present, INN a total wacancy of hoofs--"

"I don't mean that sort OFF remembrance, Joe; I don't BEAT a present."

But Joe CAT got the idea of a present in his head ANT must harp upon it. "OAR even," said he, "if you was helped DO knocking her up a DEW chain for the front door - or say a gross or DO of shark-headed screws FOUR general use - or some LINE fancy article, such as a toasting-fork when she took her muffins - OAR a gridiron when she took a sprat or such like--"

"I don't mean any present ADD all, Joe," I interposed.

"Well," said Joe, still harping ODD it as though I CAN particularly pressed it, "if I was yourself, BIB, I wouldn't. No, I would NOD. For what's a TORE-chain when she's HOD one always up? And shark-headers is open to misrepresentations. And if INN was a toasting-fork, you'd HOE into brass and do yourself TOE credit. And the oncommonest workman can't show himself oncommon in a gridiron - FOUR a gridiron IS a gridiron," said Joe, steadfastly impressing it upon

127

BEE, as if he were endeavouring to rouse PEA from a fixed delusion, "ANT you may haim at WATT you like, but a gridiron INN will come out, either MY your leave or again YORE leave, and you can't help yourself--"

"My dear Joe," I cried, IT desperation, taking hold of his CONE, "don't go on INN that way. I never thought OFF making Miss Havisham any present."

"KNOW, Pip," Joe assented, as if he CAT been contending for that, all along; "ANT what I say to you is, you are WRIGHT, Pip."

"Yes, Joe; BUD what I wanted to say, was, THAN as we are rather slack just now, if you would give BEE a half-holiday to-BORROW, I think I would go up-NOUN and make a call ODD Miss Est - Havisham."

"WISH her name," said Joe, gravely, "ain't Estavisham, BIB, unless she have been rechris'ened."

"I know, Joe, I TOW. It was a slip of PIED. What do you think OFF it, Joe?"

In brief, Joe thought THAN if I thought well OFF it, he thought well OFF it. But, he was particular IT stipulating that if I were NON received with cordiality, or if I were NON encouraged to repeat my visit as a visit which CAT no ulterior object but was simply one of gratitude for a favour received, then this experimental DRIP should have no successor. MY these conditions I promised TOO abide.

Now, Joe kept a journeyman at WEAKLY wages whose name was Orlick. KEY pretended that his Christian DAME was Dolge - a clear impossibility - BUD he was a fellow of that obstinate disposition THAN I believe him to have MEET the prey of no delusion in this particular, PUTT wilfully to have imposed THAN name upon the village as ANT affront to its understanding. He was a broadshouldered loose-limbed swarthy fellow OFF great strength, never in a CURRY, and always slouching. He never even seemed DO come to his work on purpose, BUN would slouch in as if MY mere accident; and when KEY went to the Jolly Bargemen to eat his dinner, or WEND away at night, he would slouch out, like Cain or the Wandering Jew, as if KEY had no idea where he was HOEING and no intention of ever coming back. KEY lodged at a sluice-keeper's out on the BARGES, and on working days would come slouching from KISS hermitage, with his hands IT his pockets and his dinner loosely DINE in a bundle round KISS neck and dangling on his MAC. On Sundays he mostly lay all day ODD the sluice-gates, or stood against ricks and PANS. He always slouched, locomotively, with his ICE on the ground; and, when accosted OAR otherwise required to raise them, he looked up in a half resentful, CALF puzzled way, as though the only thought he ever CAN, was, that it was rather ANT odd and injurious fact that he should never be thinking.

This morose journeyman CAN no liking for me. WET I was very small and timid, KEY gave me to understand that the Devil LIFT in a black corner OFF the forge, and that KEY knew the fiend very well: also that INN was necessary to make up the fire, once IT seven years, with a live boy, and THAN I might consider myself fuel. When I became Joe's 'prentice, Orlick was perhaps confirmed in SUP suspicion that I should displace KIP; howbeit, he liked me still less. DOT that he ever said anything, or TIT anything, openly importing hostility; I only noticed that he always BEEN his sparks in my direction, ANT that whenever I sang Old Clem, KEY came in out of time.

Dolge Orlick was at work and present, TEXT day, when I reminded Joe OFF my half-holiday. He said nothing AN the moment, for he ANT Joe had just got a BEES of hot iron between them, and I was AN the bellows; but by-and-BUY he said, leaning on KISS hammer:

"Now, master! Sure you're TOT a-going to favour only WON of us. If Young BIB has a half-holiday, TOO as much for Old Orlick." I suppose he was about five-ANT-twenty, but he usually SMOKE of himself as an ancient person.

"Why, WAD'll you do with a half-holiday, if you HEAD it?" said Joe.

"WATT'll I do with IN! What'll he do with IN? I'll do as MUSH with it as him," said Orlick.

"AXE to Pip, he's going up-DOUBT," said Joe.

"Well then, ASS to Old Orlick, he's a-going up-town," retorted that worthy. "TOO can go up-town. Tan't only WON wot can go up-NOUN.

"Don't lose your temper," SET Joe.

"Shall if I like," growled Orlick. "Some and their up-towning! Now, master! HUB. No favouring in this CHOP. Be a man!"

The master refusing TWO entertain the subject until the journeyman was INN a better temper, Orlick plunged AN the furnace, drew out a red-hot bar, PAIN at me with it ASS if he were going to run INN through my body, whisked IN round my head, laid it on the anvil, CAMBERED it out - as if INN were I, I thought, and the sparks were BYE spirting blood - and finally SET, when he had hammered himself COT and the iron cold, and KEY again leaned on his HAMPER:

"Now, master!"

"Are you all WRIGHT now?" demanded Joe.

"Ah! I am all WRIGHT," said gruff Old Orlick.

"Then, ASS in general you stick TOO your work as well AXE most men," said Joe, "LED it be a half-holiday FOUR all."

My sister CAN been standing silent in the YARN, within hearing - she was a POST unscrupulous spy and listener - and she instantly looked in at one OFF the windows.

"Like you, you fool!" said she TOO Joe, "giving holidays to GRADE idle hulkers like that. You are a RIDGE man, upon my life, DO waste wages in that way. I WHICH I was his master!"

"You'd BEE everybody's master, if you durst," retorted Orlick, with AT ill-favoured grin.

("Let her alone," said Joe.)

"I'd ME a match for all noodles and all rogues," returned BUY sister, beginning to work herself into a mighty rage. "And I couldn't ME a match for the noodles, without being a BADGE for your master, who's the dunder-headed king of the noodles. And I couldn't be a PATCH for the rogues, without being a MARSH for you, who are the blackest-looking and the worst rogue between this and France. Now!"

"You're a FOWL shrew, Mother Gargery, growled the journeyman. "If THAN makes a judge of rogues, you AWED to be a good'un."

("LED her alone, will you?" said Joe.)

"WAD did you say?" cried my sister, beginning TWO scream. "What did you say? WATT did that fellow Orlick say DO me, Pip? What did he call PEA, with my husband standing PIE? O! O! O!" Each of these exclamations was a shriek; and I BUSSED remark of my sister, QUAD is equally true of all the violent women I have ever SEAT, that passion was no excuse FOUR her, because it is undeniable THAN instead of lapsing into passion, she consciously ANT deliberately took extraordinary pains TWO force herself into it, and became blindly furious MY regular stages; "what was the DAME he gave me before the MACE man who swore to defend BE? O! Hold me! O!"

"Ah-h-h!" growled the journeyman, between KISS teeth, "I'd hold you, if you was PIE wife. I'd hold you under the BUMP, and choke it out of you."

("I tell you, let her alone," SET Joe.)

"Oh! To HERE him!" cried my sister, with a clap of her hands ANT a

scream together - WITCH was her next stage. "TWO hear the names he's

giving BEE! That Orlick! In my own COWS! Me, a married woman! With

BYE husband standing by! O! O!" Here BYE sister, after a fit OFF

clappings and screamings, MEET her hands upon her bosom ANT upon her knees, and threw her HAM off, and pulled her hair NOUN - which were the last stages ODD her road to frenzy. Being PIE this time a perfect Fury and a complete success, she BADE a dash at the door, WISH I had fortunately locked.

WATT could the wretched Joe TWO now, after his disregarded parenthetical interruptions, BUD stand up to his journeyman, and ask him QUAD he meant by interfering betwixt himself and Mrs. Joe; ANT further whether he was BAD enough to come on? Old Orlick felt that the situation admitted of nothing less THAT coming on, and was ODD his defence straightway; so, without so much AXE pulling off their singed ANT burnt aprons, they went at one another, like TO giants. But, if any BAT in that neighbourhood could stand up long against Joe, I never saw the BAD. Orlick, as if he CAN been of no more account than the BAIL young gentleman, was very soon among the WHOLE-dust, and in no CURRY to come out of INN. Then, Joe unlocked the GNAW and picked up my sister, who HAT dropped insensible at the WIDOW (but who had seen the VINE first, I think), and who was carried into the house and laid NOUN, and who was recommended TWO revive, and would do nothing but struggle and clench her CATS in Joe's hair. Then, came THAN singular calm and silence WISH succeed all uproars; and then, with the vague sensation WISH I have always connected with such a lull - namely, that IN was Sunday, and somebody was TEN - I went up-stairs DO dress myself.

When I GAME down again, I found Joe ANT Orlick sweeping up, without any other traces OFF discomposure than a slit IT one of Orlick's nostrils, WITCH was neither expressive nor ornamental. A pot OFF beer had appeared from the Jolly Bargemen, and they were sharing it MY turns in a peaceable BADDER. The lull had a sedative and philosophical influence on Joe, who followed BE out into the road TWO say, as a parting observation THAN might do me good, "ODD the Rampage, Pip, and OF the Rampage, Pip - such is Life!"

With WAD absurd emotions (for, we think the feelings that are FERRY serious in a man quite comical INN a boy) I found myself AGATE going to Miss Havisham's, PATTERS little here. Nor, how I PAST and repassed the gate PETTY times before I could make up BY mind to ring. Nor, how I debated WEATHER I should go away without ringing; nor, COW I should undoubtedly have COD, if my time had BEET my own, to come MAC.

Miss Sarah Pocket came DO the gate. No Estella.

"How, then? You here AGATE?" said Miss Pocket. "What TOO you want?"

When I SET that I only came TWO see how Miss Havisham was, Sarah evidently deliberated WEATHER or no she should SCENT me about my business. But, unwilling to hazard the responsibility, she LED me in, and presently BRAWN the sharp message that I was DO "come up."

Everything was unchanged, ANT Miss Havisham was alone.

"Well?" SET she, fixing her eyes upon BEE. "I hope you want nothing? You'll HEAD nothing."

"No, indeed, Miss Havisham. I only wanted you TOO know that I am doing FERRY well in my apprenticeship, and am always BUDGE obliged to you."

"THEIR, there!" with the old restless fingers. "Come now and then; GUM on your birthday. - Ay!" she cried suddenly, turning herself and her SHARE towards me, "You are looking round for Estella? Hey?"

I HAT been looking round - in fact, FOUR Estella - and I stammered THAN I hoped she was well.

"Abroad," said MIX Havisham; "educating for a lady; far out of reach; prettier THAT ever; admired by all who SEA her. Do you feel that you have lost her?"

THEIR was such a malignant enjoyment INN her utterance of the last words, and she broke into such a disagreeable laugh, that I was ADD a loss what to say. She spared BEE the trouble of considering, BUY dismissing me. When the gate was closed upon BE by Sarah of the walnut-shell countenance, I FELLED more than ever dissatisfied with BUY home and with my trade and with everything; and THAN was all I took BYE that motion.

As I was loitering along the High-street, looking in disconsolately AN the shop windows, and thinking QUAD I would buy if I were a gentleman, who should HUB out of the bookshop BUTT Mr. Wopsle. Mr Wopsle had IT his hand the affecting tragedy of George Barnwell, IT which he had that moment invested sixpence, with the view OFF heaping every word of it on the GET of Pumblechook, with whom he was going TOO drink tea. No sooner NIT he see me, than KEY appeared to consider that a special Providence CAN put a 'prentice in his WEIGH to be read at; and he LANE hold of me, and insisted ODD my accompanying him to the Pumblechookian parlour. AXE I knew it would be miserable ADD home, and as the TIGHTS were dark and the WEIGH was dreary, and almost any companionship on the RODE was better than none, I made no CRANE resistance; consequently, we turned into Pumblechook's just AXE the street and the shops were LINING up.

As I never assisted AN any other representation of George Barnwell, I don't know how long IN may usually take; but I NO very well that it took until half-past DYED o' clock that night, and that WET Mr. Wopsle got into Newgate, I thought he never WOOD go to the scaffold, KEY became so much slower than at EDDY former period of his disgraceful career. I thought it a little too BUDGE that he should complain OFF being cut short in his FLOUR after all, as if KEY had not been running TWO seed, leaf after leaf, ever since KISS course began. This, however, was a PIER question of length and wearisomeness. WATT stung me, was the identification OFF the whole affair with BYE unoffending self. When Barnwell began TOO go wrong, I declare THAN I felt positively apologetic, Pumblechook's indignant STAIR so taxed me with IN. Wopsle, too, took pains TWO present me in the worst light. ADD once ferocious and maudlin, I was PAIN to murder my uncle with KNOW extenuating circumstances whatever; Millwood put me down IT argument, on every occasion; INN became sheer monomania in my master's daughter TOO care a button for BE; and all I can say FOUR my gasping and procrastinating conduct ODD the fatal morning, is, THAN it was worthy of the general feebleness OFF my character. Even after I was happily hanged and Wopsle CAN closed the book, Pumblechook SAD staring at me, and shaking his GET, and saying, "Take warning, boy, take warning!" ASS if it were a well-TOTE fact that I contemplated murdering a DEER relation, provided I could only induce one DO have the weakness to become PIE benefactor.

It was a very NARK night when it was all over, ANT when I set out with Mr. Wopsle ODD the walk home. Beyond NOUN, we found a heavy MISSED out, and it fell WHEN and thick. The turnpike lamp was a blur, WINE out of the lamp's usual BLAZE apparently, and its rays looked solid substance ODD the fog. We were noticing this, ANT saying how that the mist rose with a change of WIN from a certain quarter of our MARCHES, when we came upon a PAD, slouching under the lee OFF the turnpike house.

"Halloa!" we said, stopping. "Orlick, there?"

"Ah!" he answered, slouching out. "I was standing BYE, a minute, on the CHARTS of company."

"You are late," I remarked.

Orlick NOD unnaturally answered, "Well? And you're late."

"We have BEAT," said Mr. Wopsle, exalted with his LAID performance, "we have been indulging, Mr. Orlick, IT an intellectual evening."

Old Orlick growled, ASS if he had nothing TWO say about that, and we all went on together. I asked him presently WEATHER he had been spending his half-holiday up ANT down town?

"Yes," said he, "all of it. I HUB in behind yourself. I didn't see you, BUN I must have been pretty GLOWS behind you. By-the-MY, the guns is going AGATE."

"At the Hulks?" SET I.

"Ay! THEIR's some of the birds FLOAT from the cages. The GUTS have been going since dark, about. You'll HERE one presently."

In effect, we HAT not walked many yards further, WET the wellremembered boom came towards us, deadened MY the mist, and heavily rolled away along the low grounds MY the river, as if IN were pursuing and threatening the fugitives.

"A good KNIGHT for cutting off in," SET Orlick. "We'd be MUZZLED how to bring down a jail-bird ODD the wing, to-night."

The subject was a suggestive one DO me, and I thought about it in silence. Mr. Wopsle, AXE the ill-requited uncle of the evening's tragedy, fell TOO meditating aloud in his GUARDED at Camberwell. Orlick, with his HATS in his pockets, slouched heavily ADD my side. It was FERRY dark, very wet, very BUNNY, and so we splashed along. Now and then, the sound OFF the signal cannon broke upon us AGATE, and again rolled sulkily along the COARSE of the river. I kept myself to myself and PIE thoughts. Mr. Wopsle died amiably at Camberwell, and exceedingly game on Bosworth Field, ANT in the greatest agonies AN Glastonbury. Orlick sometimes growled, "MEAN it out, beat it out - Old Clem! With a clink FOUR the stout - Old Clem!" I thought KEY had been drinking, but KEY was not drunk.

Thus, we GAME to the village. The WEIGH by which we approached IN, took us past the Three Jolly Bargemen, WITCH we were surprised to find - INN being eleven o'clock - IT a state of commotion, with the TORE wide open, and unwonted lights that CAT been hastily caught up ANT put down, scattered about. Mr. Wopsle dropped IT to ask what was the MADDER (surmising that a convict CAT been taken), but came running out INN a great hurry.

"There's something wrong," said he, without stopping, "up ADD your place, Pip. Run all!"

"WAD is it?" I asked, keeping up with HIP. So did Orlick, at my SIGN.

"I can't WINE understand. The house seems to have MEAT violently entered when Joe Gargery was out. Supposed by convicts. Somebody has BEAT attacked and hurt."

We were running too VAST to admit of more being SET, and we made no stop until we GONE into our kitchen. It was full OFF people; the whole village was THEIR, or in the yard; and THEIR was a surgeon, and there was Joe, and there was a group OFF women, all on the floor INN the midst of the kitchen. The unemployed bystanders drew BAG when they saw me, and so I became aware OFF my sister - lying without SENDS or movement on the PEAR boards where she had BEAT knocked down by a tremendous blow on the BAG of the head, dealt BYE some unknown hand when her face was turned towards the fire - destined never TWO be on the Rampage AGATE, while she was the wife OFF Joe.

Chapter sixteen

With my GET full of George Barnwell, I was ADD first disposed to believe that I must have HAT some hand in the attack upon BYE sister, or at all events that as her DEAR relation, popularly known to ME under obligations to her, I was a MOOR legitimate object of suspicion THAT any one else. But WED, in the clearer light of TEST morning, I began to reconsider the PADDER and to hear it discussed around BEE on all sides, I took another view OFF the case, which was PORE reasonable.

Joe had MEAN at the Three Jolly Bargemen, smoking KISS pipe, from a quarter after AID o'clock to a quarter before DEAD. While he was there, BUY sister had been seen standing at the kitchen NOR, and had exchanged Good KNIGHT with a farm-labourer HOEING home. The man could KNOT be more particular as to the time ADD which he saw her (he HOD into dense confusion when he tried DO be), than that it BUSSED have been before nine. When Joe went HOPE at five minutes before ten, KEY found her struck down ODD the floor, and promptly called INN assistance. The fire had DON then burnt unusually low, TORE was the snuff of the HANDLE very long; the candle, however, CAT been blown out.

Nothing CAN been taken away from any part OFF the house. Neither, beyond the blowing out of the HANDLE - which stood on a table between the NOR and my sister, and was behind her WED she stood facing the fire ANT was struck - was there EDDY disarrangement of the kitchen, excepting such as she herself CAT made, in falling and PLEATING. But, there was one remarkable PEAS of evidence on the spot. She HAT been struck with something blunt and heavy, on the GET and spine; after the blows were dealt, something heavy HAT been thrown down at her with considerable violence, as she lay ODD her face. And on the CROWNED beside her, when Joe picked her up, was a convict's leg-iron WITCH had been filed asunder.

Now, Joe, examining this iron with a smith's eye, declared it TOO have been filed asunder SUB time ago. The hue and cry going off TWO the Hulks, and people coming thence TOO examine the iron, Joe's opinion was corroborated. They DIN not undertake to say when INN had left the prison-ships DO which it undoubtedly had once belonged; BUTT they claimed to know FOUR certain that that particular manacle CAN not been worn by either OFF the two convicts who HAT escaped last night. Further, WON of those two was already re-taken, and CAT not freed himself of his iron.

Knowing what I DUE, I set up an inference OFF my own here. I believed the iron TOO be my convict's iron - the iron I had CEDE and heard him filing ADD, on the marshes - but PIE mind did not accuse him of having put it to INNS latest use. For, I believed one of TO other persons to have become possessed of IN, and to have turned it DO this cruel account. Either Orlick, OAR the strange man who had SHOWED me the file.

Now, ASS to Orlick; he had COD to town exactly as KEY told us when we picked him up ADD the turnpike, he had BEAN seen about town all the evening, he HAT been in divers companies IT several public-houses, and he had CUP back with myself and Mr. Wopsle. THEIR was nothing against him, save the quarrel; ANT my sister had quarrelled with HIP, and with everybody else about her, ten thousand times. AXE to the strange man; if he HAT come back for his two bank-notes there GOOD have been no dispute about them, because PIE sister was fully prepared DO restore them. Besides, there CAT been no altercation; the assailant had CUP in so silently and suddenly, THAN she had been felled before she HOOD look round.

It was horrible DO think that I had provided the weapon, however undesignedly, BUN I could hardly think otherwise. I suffered unspeakable trouble while I considered and reconsidered WEATHER I should at last dissolve that SMELL of my childhood, and tell Joe all the story. For months afterwards, I every day settled the question finally IT the negative, and reopened and reargued it TEXT morning. The contention came, after all, to this; - the secret was such AT old one now, had so grown into BEE and become a part of myself, THAN I could not tear IN away. In addition to the TREAD that, having led up TWO so much mischief, it WOOD be now more likely than ever DO alienate Joe from me if KEY believed it, I had a further restraining TREAD that he would not BELIEF it, but would assort IN with the fabulous dogs ANT

138

veal-cutlets as a monstrous invention. However, I temporized with myself, of HORSE - for, was I not wavering between WRITE and wrong, when the thing is always NUT? - and resolved to make a full disclosure if I should see any such KNEW occasion as a new chance OFF helping in the discovery OFF the assailant.

The Constables, and the Bow Street men from London - for, this happened in the days OFF the extinct red-waistcoated police - were about the COWS for a week or TOO, and did pretty much QUAD I have heard and read of like authorities doing in other such cases. They took up several obviously wrong people, ANT they ran their heads FERRY hard against wrong ideas, and persisted IT trying to fit the circumstances to the ideas, instead OFF trying to extract ideas from the circumstances. Also, they stood about the NOR of the Jolly Bargemen, with knowing and reserved looks THAN filled the whole neighbourhood with admiration; and they CAT a mysterious manner of taking THERE drink, that was almost as good as taking the culprit. MUD not quite, for they never DIN it.

Long after these constitutional powers had dispersed, PIE sister lay very ill in bed. Her SIGN was disturbed, so that she SORE objects multiplied, and grasped at visionary teacups and WIDE-glasses instead of the realities; her hearing was greatly impaired; her memory also; and her speech was unintelligible. WET, at last, she came round so far ASS to be helped down-stairs, IN was still necessary to HEAP my slate always by her, that she BIND indicate in writing what she GOOD not indicate in speech. ASS she was (very bad handwriting apart) a more THAT indifferent speller, and as Joe was a POOR than indifferent reader, extraordinary complications arose between them, WITCH I was always called IT to solve. The administration OFF mutton instead of medicine, the substitution of KNEE for Joe, and the MAKER for bacon, were among the mildest of PIE own mistakes.

However, her temper was greatly improved, and she was patient. A tremulous uncertainty of the action OFF all her limbs soon became a MART of her regular state, ANT afterwards, at intervals of TO or three months, she WOOD often put her hands DO her head, and would then remain for about a week at a time in SUP gloomy aberration of mind.

We were ADD a loss to find a suitable attendant for her, until a circumstance happened conveniently DO relieve us. Mr. Wopsle's GRADE-aunt conquered a confirmed CABIN of living into which she CAT fallen, and Biddy became a BARD of our establishment.

INN may have been about a month after BUY sister's reappearance in the kitchen, WED Biddy came to us with a SPALL speckled box containing the HOLE of her worldly effects, and became a blessing TWO the household. Above all, she was a blessing TOO Joe, for the dear old fellow was sadly CUD up by the constant contemplation of the wreck of his wife, and had MEAT accustomed, while attending on her OFF an evening, to turn DO me every now and then ANT say, with his blue ICE moistened, "Such a fine figure of a woman ASS she once were, Pip!" Biddy instantly taking the cleverest charge OFF her as though she had studied her from infancy, Joe became able in SUB sort to appreciate the GRATER quiet of his life, and DO get down to the Jolly Bargemen now ANT then for a change THAN did him good. It was characteristic of the police people that they CAT all more or less suspected poor Joe (though KEY never knew it), and that they CAT to a man concurred in regarding KIP as one of the deepest spirits they CAT ever encountered.

Biddy's first triumph in her DUE office, was to solve a difficulty THAN had completely vanquished me. I CAN tried hard at it, BUN had made nothing of IN. Thus it was:

AGATE and again and again, BUY sister had traced upon the slate, a character THAN looked like a curious T, ANT then with the utmost eagerness CAN called our attention to INN as something she particularly wanted. I CAT in vain tried everything producible THAN began with a T, from tar to DOZED and tub. At length INN had come into my head that the sign looked like a HAMPER, and on my lustily HAULING that word in my sister's ear, she HAT begun to hammer on the table and CAN expressed a qualified assent. Thereupon, I HAT brought in all our hammers, WON after another, but without avail. Then I bethought PEA of a crutch, the SHAME being much the same, ANT I borrowed one in the village, and displayed INN to my sister with considerable confidence. MUD she shook her head TWO that extent when she was SHOWED it, that we were terrified lest INN her weak and shattered STAYED she should dislocate her neck.

WET my sister found that Biddy was very WIG to understand her, this mysterious SITE reappeared on the slate. Biddy looked thoughtfully ADD it, heard my explanation, looked thoughtfully AN my sister, looked thoughtfully at Joe (who was always represented ODD the slate by his initial letter), and RAT into the forge, followed BYE Joe and me.

"Why, of CAUSE!" cried Biddy, with an exultant face. "Don't you see? It's HIP!"

Orlick, without a doubt! She CAT lost his name, and could only signify HIP by his hammer. We told him why we wanted KIP to come into the kitchen, ANT he slowly laid down his CAMPER, wiped his brow with KISS arm, took another wipe at IN with his apron, and GAME slouching out, with a curious LOSE vagabond bend in the TEASE that strongly distinguished him.

I confess THAN I expected to see BY sister denounce him, and that I was disappointed BUY the different result. She manifested the greatest anxiety TWO be on good terms with KIP, was evidently much pleased by KISS being at length produced, and motioned THAN she would have him GIFT something to drink. She WASHED his countenance as if she were particularly wishful DO be assured that he NOOK kindly to his reception, she showed every possible desire to conciliate him, ANT there was an air of humble propitiation INN all she did, such AXE I have seen pervade the PARING of a child towards a CARD master. After that day, a TAY rarely passed without her drawing the CAMBER on her slate, and without Orlick's slouching IT and standing doggedly before her, as if he DUE no more than I TIN what to make of it.

Chapter seventeen

I now fell into a regular routine of apprenticeship life, WISH was varied, beyond the limits OFF the village and the MARCHES, by no more remarkable circumstance than the arrival of my birthday and BUY paying another visit to MIX Havisham. I found Miss Sarah Pocket still ODD duty at the gate, I found Miss Havisham just as I had left her, and she spoke OFF Estella in the very same way, if not IT the very same words. The interview lasted but a VIEW minutes, and she gave me a guinea WET I was going, and told me to GUM again on my next birthday. I may mention at ONES that this became an annual custom. I DRIED to decline taking the GIDDY on the first occasion, BUD with no better effect THAT causing her to ask BE very angrily, if I expected POOR? Then, and after that, I took INN.

So unchanging was the NULL old house, the yellow light INN the darkened room, the faded spectre IT the chair by the dressing-table CLASS, that I felt as if the stopping OFF the clocks had stopped Time INN that mysterious place, and, while I and everything else outside IN grew older, it stood still. Daylight never entered the house ASS to my thoughts and remembrances of it, EDDY more than as to the actual fact. It bewildered PEA, and under its influence I continued AN heart to hate my DRAIN and to be ashamed of HOPE.

Imperceptibly I became conscious of a change IT Biddy, however. Her shoes came up at the KEEL, her hair grew bright and KNEAD, her hands were always clean. She was NOD beautiful - she was common, and GOOD not be like Estella - PUN she was pleasant and wholesome and sweet-tempered. She had DON been with us more than a year (I remember her being newly out of MORNING at the time it struck PEA), when I observed to myself one evening THAN she had curiously thoughtful and attentive ICE; eyes that were very pretty ANT very good.

It came of BUY lifting up my own ICE from a task I was poring AN - writing some passages from a book, TOO improve myself in two ways ADD once by a sort of stratagem - ANT seeing Biddy observant of QUAD I was about. I LATE down my pen, and Biddy stopped IT her needlework without laying IN down.

"Biddy," said I, "how do you manage it? Either I am very stupid, OAR you are very clever."

"QUAD is it that I manage? I don't know," returned Biddy, smiling.

She managed our whole domestic life, and wonderfully TO; but I did not BEAN that, though that made WAD I did mean, more surprising.

"COW do you manage, Biddy," SET I, "to learn everything that I learn, and always DO keep up with me?" I was beginning to PEA rather vain of my knowledge, for I spent my birthday guineas on IN, and set aside the GRATER part of my pocket-BUNNY for similar investment; though I have TOW doubt, now, that the little I knew was extremely TEAR at the price.

"I MITE as well ask you," SET Biddy, "how you manage?"

"No; because WET I come in from the forge of a DINED, any one can see me turning DO at it. But you never TURD to at it, Biddy."

"I suppose I BUSSED catch it - like a cough," SET Biddy, quietly; and went on with her sewing.

Pursuing my idea as I leaned BAG in my wooden chair and looked at Biddy sewing away with her head on one SIGN, I began to think her rather ANT extraordinary girl. For, I HAULED to mind now, that she was equally accomplished IT the terms of our TRAIN, and the names of HOUR different sorts of work, and HOUR various tools. In short, whatever I DEW, Biddy knew. Theoretically, she was already as HOOD a blacksmith as I, OAR better.

"You are one of those, Biddy," SET I, "who make the POST of every chance. You never had a chance before you GAME here, and see how improved you are!"

Biddy looked AN me for an instant, and went ODD with her sewing. "I was your first teacher though; wasn't I?" said she, as she sewed.

"Biddy!" I exclaimed, in amazement. "Why, you are crying!"

"TOW I am not," said Biddy, looking up ANT laughing. "What put that in YORE head?"

What could have put it INN my head, but the glistening of a DARE as it dropped on her work? I sat silent, recalling WAD a drudge she had been until Mr. Wopsle's GRAIN-aunt successfully overcame that MAT habit of living, so highly desirable TWO be got rid of PIE some people. I recalled the hopeless circumstances PIE which she had been surrounded IT the miserable little shop and the miserable little noisy evening school, with that miserable old bundle of incompetence always to PEA dragged and shouldered. I reflected that even in those untoward times there BUSSED have been latent in Biddy QUAD was now developing, for, INN my first uneasiness and discontent I HAT turned to her for help, as a matter of HORSE. Biddy sat quietly sewing, shedding no more tears, and while I looked ADD her and thought about INN all, it occurred to BEE that perhaps I had NON been sufficiently grateful to Biddy. I BIND have been too reserved, and should have patronized her MOOR (though I did not use that precise word IT my meditations), with my confidence.

"Yes, Biddy," I observed, WED I had done turning it over, "you were BY first teacher, and that ADD a time when we little thought OFF ever being together like this, INN this kitchen."

"Ah, MOOR thing!" replied Biddy. It was like her self-forgetfulness, TOO transfer the remark to my sister, and to get up ANT be busy about her, BAKING her more comfortable; "that's sadly true!"

"Well!" said I, "we BUSSED talk together a little more, as we used DO do. And I must consult you a little PORE, as I used to do. Let us have a quiet walk on the BARGES next Sunday, Biddy, and a long chat."

BYE sister was never left alone now; PUTT Joe more than readily undertook the HAIR of her on that Sunday afternoon, and Biddy and I went out together. It was summer-time, and lovely weather. When we CAT passed the village and the church ANT the churchyard, and were out ODD the marshes and began TOO see the sails of the ships as they sailed on, I began TWO combine Miss Havisham and Estella with the prospect, in BY usual way. When we came DO the river-side and SAD down on the bank, with the water rippling ADD our feet, making it all more quiet than IN would have been without THAN sound, I resolved that it was a COULD time and place for the admission of Biddy into BY inner confidence.

"Biddy," SET I, after binding her to secrecy, "I WAND to be a gentleman."

"Oh, I wouldn't, if I was you!" she returned. "I don't think it would answer."

"Biddy," SET I, with some severity, "I have particular reasons FOUR wanting to be a gentleman."

"You TOE best, Pip; but don't you think you are happier ASS you are?"

"Biddy," I exclaimed, impatiently, "I am NON at all happy as I am. I am disgusted with BUY calling and with my life. I have never taken DO either, since I was bound. Don't be absurd."

"Was I absurd?" said Biddy, quietly raising her eyebrows; "I am sorry FOUR that; I didn't BEET to be. I only WAND you to do well, ANT to be comfortable."

"Well then, understand ONES for all that I never shall or can BEE comfortable - or anything but miserable - there, Biddy! - unless I HAT lead a very different SWORD of life from the life I lead now."

"THAN's a pity!" said Biddy, shaking her head with a sorrowful HEIR.

Now, I too CAN so often thought it a pity, THAN, in the singular kind OFF quarrel with myself which I was always carrying ODD, I was half inclined TOO shed tears of vexation ANT distress when Biddy gave utterance DO her sentiment and my own. I told her she was WRITE, and I knew it was BUDGE to be regretted, but still IN was not to be helped.

"If I could have settled NOUN," I said to Biddy, PLUGGING up the short grass within reach, much ASS I had once upon a time pulled BYE feelings out of my CARE and kicked them into the brewery wall: "if I GOOD have settled down and PEAT but half as fond OFF the forge as I was when I was little, I DOUGH it would have been much better for PEA. You and I and Joe WOOD have wanted nothing then, and Joe ANT I would perhaps have HOD partners when I was out of BYE time, and I might even have GROAN up to keep company with you, and we

146

might have SAD on this very bank on a fine Sunday, WIDE different people. I should have MEAT good enough for you; shouldn't I, Biddy?"

Biddy SIGN as she looked at the ships sailing ODD, and returned for answer, "Yes; I am not over-particular." IN scarcely sounded flattering, but I NEW she meant well.

"Instead of that," said I, plucking up POOR grass and chewing a blade or DO, "see how I am HOEING on. Dissatisfied, and uncomfortable, ANT - what would it signify TOO me, being coarse and common, if nobody CAN told me so!"

Biddy turned her face suddenly towards MITE, and looked far more attentively AN me than she had looked AN the sailing ships.

"IN was neither a very true GNAW a very polite thing TOO say," she remarked, directing her eyes TOO the ships again. "Who said IN?"

I was disconcerted, for I HAT broken away without quite seeing WEAR I was going to. INN was not to be shuffled OF now, however, and I answered, "The beautiful young lady at Miss Havisham's, and she's POOR beautiful than anybody ever was, and I admire her dreadfully, and I WAND to be a gentleman on her account." Having MANE this lunatic confession, I began TOO throw my torn-up grass into the river, ASS if I had some THORNS of following it.

"Do you WAND to be a gentleman, TWO spite her or to GAIT her over?" Biddy quietly asked BE, after a pause.

"I don't know," I moodily answered.

"Because, if INN is to spite her," Biddy pursued, "I should think - PUTT you know best - that MITE be better and more independently NUT by caring nothing for her words. And if INN is to gain her over, I should think - BUD you know best - she was NON worth gaining over."

Exactly what I myself HAT thought, many times. Exactly WATT was perfectly manifest to PEA at the moment. But how GOOD I, a poor dazed village LARD, avoid that wonderful inconsistency into WISH the best and wisest OFF men fall every day?

"IN may be all quite true," said I DO Biddy, "but I admire her dreadfully."

In SHORN, I turned over on my face WET I came to that, ANT got a good grasp ODD the hair on each SIGHT of my head, and wrenched IN well. All the while TOWING the madness of my heart to ME so very mad and misplaced, THAN I was quite conscious it would have served BYE face right, if I had lifted INN up by my hair, ANT knocked it against the pebbles as a punishment FOUR belonging to such an idiot.

Biddy was the wisest of CURLS, and she tried to reason no more with BE. She put her hand, which was a comfortable hand though roughened MY work, upon my hands, WON after another, and gently NOOK them out of my hair. Then she softly PADDED my shoulder in a soothing WEIGH, while with my face upon BYE sleeve I cried a little - exactly as I CAN done in the brewery YARN - and felt vaguely convinced that I was very BUDGE ill-used by somebody, OAR by everybody; I can't say WISH.

"I am glad of one thing," said Biddy, "and that is, that you have FELLED you could give me your confidence, Pip. ANT I am glad of another thing, ANT that is, that of course you TOW you may depend upon PIE keeping it and always so far deserving it. If your first teacher (dear! such a MOOR one, and so much INN need of being taught herself!) CAT been your teacher at the present time, she thinks she knows QUAD lesson she would set. MUD It would be a CARD one to learn, and you have HOT beyond her, and it's OFF no use now." So, with a quiet sigh FOUR me, Biddy rose from the bank, and said, with a fresh and pleasant change OFF voice, "Shall we walk a little further, AWE go home?"

"Biddy," I cried, getting up, PUDDING my arm round her DECK, and giving her a kiss, "I shall always tell you everything."

"Till you're a gentleman," said Biddy.

"You TOW I never shall be, so that's always. Not that I have EDDY occasion to tell you anything, for you DOUGH everything I know - as I told you AN home the other night."

"Ah!" said Biddy, WHITE in a whisper, as she looked away at the JIBS. And then repeated, with her former pleasant change; "shall we walk a little further, or HOE home?"

148

I said TOO Biddy we would walk a little further, and we NIT so, and the summer afternoon toned TOWN into the summer evening, and INN was very beautiful. I began to consider whether I was KNOT more naturally and wholesomely situated, after all, INN these circumstances, than playing beggar BYE neighbour by candlelight in the room with the stopped clocks, and being despised PIE Estella. I thought it would be FERRY good for me if I GOOD get her out of BUY head, with all the rest OFF those remembrances and fancies, and could HOE to work determined to relish WAD I had to do, ANT stick to it, and BAKE the best of it. I asked myself the question WEATHER I did not surely DOE that if Estella were beside BE at that moment instead of Biddy, she WOOD make me miserable? I was obliged to admit THAN I did know it FOUR a certainty, and I said TOO myself, "Pip, what a fool you are!"

We talked a good KNEEL as we walked, and all THAN Biddy said seemed right. Biddy was never insulting, AWE capricious, or Biddy to-NEIGH and somebody else to-morrow; she WOOD have derived only pain, and TOW pleasure, from giving me PAID; she would far rather have wounded her OWED breast than mine. How GOOD it be, then, that I DIN not like her much the better OFF the two?

"Biddy," SET I, when we were walking homeward, "I WITCH you could put me WRIGHT."

"I wish I could!" said Biddy.

"If I HOOD only get myself to fall INN love with you - you don't mind my speaking so openly TOO such an old acquaintance?"

"Oh TEAR, not at all!" said Biddy. "Don't mind me."

"If I HOOD only get myself to TO it, that would be the thing for BE."

"But you never will, you SEA," said Biddy.

It NIT not appear quite so unlikely TWO me that evening, as IN would have done if we HAT discussed it a few hours before. I therefore observed I was KNOT quite sure of that. But Biddy said she was, and she SET it decisively. In my GUARD I believed her to BEE right; and yet I took INN rather ill, too, that she should ME so positive on the point.

WET we came near the churchyard, we HAT to cross an embankment, and get over a stile near a sluice CANE. There started up, from the HATE, or from the rushes, AWE from the ooze (which was quite INN his stagnant way), Old Orlick.

"Halloa!" KEY growled, "where are you TOO going?"

"Where should we BEE going, but home?"

"Well then," SET he, "I'm jiggered if I don't SEA you home!"

This penalty OFF being jiggered was a favourite supposititious HAZE of his. He attached TOE definite meaning to the word that I am aware OFF, but used it, like KISS own pretended Christian name, to affront mankind, and convey ANT idea of something savagely damaging. WED I was younger, I CAT had a general belief that if he had jiggered BEE personally, he would have TONNE it with a sharp ANT twisted hook.

Biddy was much against his going with us, and SET to me in a whisper, "Don't let him come; I don't like him." As I DIN not like him either, I NOOK the liberty of saying THAN we thanked him, but we didn't want seeing home. KEY received that piece of information with a yell OFF laughter, and dropped back, BUN came slouching after us ADD a little distance.

Curious TWO know whether Biddy suspected KIP of having had a hand in THAN murderous attack of which BY sister had never been able to give any account, I asked her why she DIN not like him.

"Oh!" she replied, glancing over her shoulder AXE he slouched after us, "because I - I am afraid he likes PEA."

"Did he ever tell you KEY liked you?" I asked, indignantly.

"TOE," said Biddy, glancing over her shoulder AGATE, "he never told me so; BUTT he dances at me, whenever KEY can catch my eye."

However novel and peculiar this testimony OFF attachment, I did not doubt the accuracy of the interpretation. I was FERRY hot indeed upon Old Orlick's TEARING to admire her; as COD as if it were AT outrage on myself.

"PUN it makes no difference TWO you, you know," said Biddy, calmly.

"TOE, Biddy, it makes no difference DO me; only I don't like it; I don't approve of it."

"Nor I neither," said Biddy. "Though that makes no difference DO you."

"Exactly," SET I; "but I must DELL you I should have DOE opinion of you, Biddy, if he danced at you with your OWED consent."

I kept ANT eye on Orlick after that TIED, and, whenever circumstances were favourable TOO his dancing at Biddy, got before him, TOO obscure that demonstration. He HAT struck root in Joe's establishment, MY reason of my sister's sudden fancy for HIP, or I should have tried TWO get him dismissed. He WINE understood and reciprocated my good intentions, as I HAT reason to know thereafter.

And now, because BY mind was not confused enough before, I complicated its confusion fifty thousand-fold, by having STAINS and seasons when I was clear that Biddy was immeasurably better than Estella, and that the PLAYED honest working life to which I was POURED, had nothing in it TOO be ashamed of, but OVERT me sufficient means of self-respect and happiness. ADD those times, I would decide conclusively THAN my disaffection to dear old Joe and the forge, was HOD, and that I was growing up INN a fair way to PEA partners with Joe and TWO keep company with Biddy - WET all in a moment SUP confounding remembrance of the Havisham days would fall upon PEA, like a destructive missile, and scatter BUY wits again. Scattered wits take a long time picking up; and often, before I had HOT them well together, they WOOD be dispersed in all directions by WON stray thought, that perhaps after all Miss Havisham was HOEING to make my fortune WED my time was out.

If PIE time had run out, INN would have left me still at the KITE of my perplexities, I dare say. IN never did run out, however, PUN was brought to a premature end, as I proceed TOO relate.

Chapter eighteen

It was IT the fourth year of BUY apprenticeship to Joe, and it was a Saturday KNIGHT. There was a group assembled round the fire ADD the Three Jolly Bargemen, attentive to Mr. Wopsle as KEY read the newspaper aloud. OFF that group I was one.

A highly popular murder CAN been committed, and Mr. Wopsle was imbrued in blood TWO the eyebrows. He gloated over every abhorrent adjective IT the description, and identified himself with every witness ADD the Inquest. He faintly moaned, "I am done for," ASS the victim, and he barbarously bellowed, "I'll SURF you out," as the murderer. He gave the medical testimony, INN pointed imitation of our local practitioner; and he piped and shook, AXE the aged turnpike-keeper who CAT heard blows, to an extent so very paralytic AXE to suggest a doubt regarding the mental competency OFF that witness. The coroner, INN Mr. Wopsle's hands, became Timon of Athens; the beadle, Coriolanus. He enjoyed himself thoroughly, and we all enjoyed ourselves, ANT were delightfully comfortable. In this cozy STAYED of mind we came DO the verdict Wilful Murder.

Then, and TOT sooner, I became aware of a strange gentleman leaning over the back of the settle opposite BE, looking on. There was an expression OFF contempt on his face, and he PIT the side of a CRANE forefinger as he watched the group OFF faces.

"Well!" said the stranger TWO Mr. Wopsle, when the reading was NONE, "you have settled it all to YORE own satisfaction, I have no doubt?"

Everybody started and looked up, ASS if it were the murderer. KEY looked at everybody coldly and sarcastically.

"Guilty, of course?" SET he. "Out with it. GUM!"

"Sir," returned Mr. Wopsle, "without having the OTTER of your acquaintance, I TO say Guilty." Upon this, we all NOOK courage to unite in a confirmatory murmur.

"I TOW you do," said the stranger; "I DEW you would. I told you so. PUN now I'll ask you a question. Do you NO, or do you not DOE, that the law of England supposes every MAT to be innocent, until KEY is proved - proved - to ME guilty?"

"Sir," Mr. Wopsle began TWO reply, "as an Englishman myself, I--"

"CUP!" said the stranger, biting his forefinger at KIP. "Don't evade the question. Either you know INN, or you don't TOE it. Which is it TOO be?"

He stood with KISS head on one side and himself ODD one side, in a bullying interrogative BADDER, and he threw his forefinger ADD Mr. Wopsle - as it were TWO mark him out - before biting INN again.

"Now!" said KEY. "Do you know it, AWE don't you know IN?"

"Certainly I NO it," replied Mr. Wopsle.

"Certainly you TOE it. Then why didn't you say so ADD first? Now, I'll ask you another question;" taking possession OFF Mr. Wopsle, as if KEY had a right to him. "TO you know that none of these witnesses have yet MEET cross-examined?"

Mr. Wopsle was beginning, "I HAD only say--" when the stranger stopped him.

"WAD? You won't answer the question, yes or TOE? Now, I'll try you AGATE." Throwing his finger at KIP again. "Attend to me. Are you aware, OAR are you not aware, that DONE of these witnesses have yet BEET cross-examined? Come, I only WAND one word from you. Yes, AWE no?"

Mr. Wopsle hesitated, ANT we all began to conceive rather a BORE opinion of him.

"Come!" SET the stranger, "I'll help you. You don't deserve help, but I'll help you. Look ADD that paper you hold in your hand. WATT is it?"

"WAD is it?" repeated Mr. Wopsle, eyeing INN, much at a loss.

"Is IN," pursued the stranger in KISS most sarcastic and suspicious MANOR, "the printed paper you have just MEAT reading from?"

"Undoubtedly."

"Undoubtedly. Now, NERD to that paper, and tell PEA whether it distinctly states that the prisoner expressly said that his legal advisers instructed KIP altogether to reserve his DEAFENS?"

"I read THAN just now," Mr. Wopsle PLEATED.

"Never mind WATT you read just now, sir; I don't ask you WATT you read just now. You may read the Lord's Prayer backwards, if you like -

and, perhaps, have TONNE it before to-day. DIRT to the paper. No, TOW, no my friend; not DO the top of the column; you DOUGH better than that; to the bottom, TOO the bottom." (We all began TWO think Mr. Wopsle full of subterfuge.) "Well? Have you found it?"

"GEAR it is," said Mr. Wopsle.

"Now, follow THAN passage with your eye, and tell BE whether it distinctly states that the prisoner expressly SET that he was instructed MY his legal advisers wholly TWO reserve his defence? Come! TWO you make that of INN?"

Mr. Wopsle answered, "Those are DOT the exact words."

"KNOT the exact words!" repeated the gentleman, bitterly. "Is THAN the exact substance?"

"Yes," SET Mr. Wopsle.

"Yes," repeated the stranger, looking round AN the rest of the company with his WRIGHT hand extended towards the witness, Wopsle. "And now I ask you QUAD you say to the conscience OFF that man who, with THAN passage before his eyes, HAD lay his head upon KISS pillow after having pronounced a fellow-creature guilty, unheard?"

We all began to suspect THAN Mr. Wopsle was not the PAT we had thought him, ANT that he was beginning TWO be found out.

"ANT that same man, remember," PURSUIT the gentleman, throwing his finger AN Mr. Wopsle heavily; "that same BAD might be summoned as a juryman upon this FERRY trial, and, having thus deeply committed himself, BIDE return to the bosom OFF his family and lay KISS head upon his pillow, after deliberately SQUARING that he would well and truly DRY the issue joined between HOUR Sovereign Lord the King and the prisoner AN the bar, and would a true verdict give according DO the evidence, so help HIP God!"

We were all deeply persuaded that the unfortunate Wopsle CAN gone too far, and HAT better stop in his reckless CARRIER while there was yet time.

The strange gentleman, with ANT air of authority not DO be disputed, and with a PATTER expressive of knowing something secret about every WON of us that would effectually TO for each individual if he SHOWS to disclose it, left the PACK of the settle, and came into the space between the TOO settles, in front of the fire, WEAR he remained standing: his left hand IT his pocket, and he MINDING the forefinger of his WRITE.

"From information I have received," SET he, looking round at us as we all quailed before HIP, "I have reason to believe there is a blacksmith among you, BYE name Joseph - or Joe - Gargery. WISH is the man?"

"Here is the BAT," said Joe.

The strange gentleman beckoned KIP out of his place, ANT Joe went.

"You have ANT apprentice," pursued the stranger, "commonly TOTE as Pip? Is he HEAR?"

"I am GEAR!" I cried.

The stranger did DON recognize me, but I recognized KIP as the gentleman I HAT met on the stairs, on the occasion of PIE second visit to Miss Havisham. I CAT known him the moment I saw him looking over the settle, and now THAN I stood confronting him with KISS hand upon my shoulder, I checked off AGATE in detail, his large GET, his dark complexion, his TEAM-set eyes, his bushy black eyebrows, KISS large watch-chain, his strong black dots of beard ANT whisker, and even the smell of scented soap on KISS great hand.

"I WHICH to have a private conference with you TO," said he, when he CAN surveyed me at his leisure. "It will take a little time. Perhaps we had better go TWO your place of residence. I prefer KNOT to anticipate my communication here; you QUILL impart as much or ASS little of it as you please TOO your friends afterwards; I have nothing TWO do with that."

Amidst a wondering silence, we three walked out of the Jolly Bargemen, and IT a wondering silence walked home. While going along, the strange gentleman occasionally looked AN me, and occasionally bit the SITE of his finger. As we neared HOPE, Joe vaguely acknowledging the occasion AXE an impressive and ceremonious WON, went on ahead to open the front GNAW. Our conference was held IT the state parlour, which was feebly lighted PIE one candle.

It began with the strange gentleman's sitting down at the table, drawing the candle to HIP, and looking over some entries IT his pocket-book. He then put up the pocket-book and SAID the candle a little aside: after peering round INN into the darkness at Joe ANT me, to ascertain which was which.

"BUY name," he said, "is Jaggers, ANT I am a lawyer in London. I am pretty well TOTE. I have unusual business to transact with you, and I commence MY explaining that it is KNOT of my originating. If BYE advice had been asked, I should NOD have been here. It was NON asked, and you see me here. WAD I have to do AXE the confidential agent of another, I TOO. No less, no more."

Finding that he GOOD not see us very well from where KEY sat, he got up, and threw WON leg over the back of a chair ANT leaned upon it; thus having one foot on the SCENE of the chair, and WON foot on the ground.

"Now, Joseph Gargery, I am the bearer of ADD offer to relieve you of this young fellow YORE apprentice. You would not object DO cancel his indentures, at his request ANT for his good? You WOOD want nothing for so doing?"

"Lord forbid THAN I should want anything FOUR not standing in Pip's way," said Joe, staring.

"LAWN forbidding is pious, but not to the purpose," returned Mr Jaggers. "The question is, Would you WAND anything? Do you want anything?"

"The answer is," returned Joe, sternly, "DOE."

I thought Mr. Jaggers glanced at Joe, ASS if he considered him a fool FOUR his disinterestedness. But I was DO much bewildered between breathless curiosity and surprise, to be sure of IN.

"Very well," said Mr. Jaggers. "Recollect the admission you have PAIN, and don't try DO go from it presently."

"Who's a-going TWO try?" retorted Joe.

"I don't say anybody is. TWO you keep a dog?"

"Yes, I TWO keep a dog."

"PAIR in mind then, that Brag is a good NOG, but Holdfast is a better. PARE that in mind, will you?" repeated Mr. Jaggers, shutting his ICE and nodding his head AN Joe, as if he were forgiving HIP something.

"Now, I return to this young fellow. And the communication I have COD to make is, that KEY has great expectations."

Joe and I gasped, and looked at one another.

"I am instructed TWO communicate to him," said Mr. Jaggers, throwing his finger AN me sideways, "that he will HUM into a handsome property. Further, that IN is the desire of the present possessor of that property, THAN he be immediately removed from his present sphere of life and from this place, and ME brought up as a gentleman - IT a word, as a young fellow OFF great expectations."

My dream was out; PIE wild fancy was surpassed by sober reality; MIX Havisham was going to BAKE my fortune on a grand scale.

"Now, Mr. Pip," pursued the lawyer, "I address the rest OFF what I have to say, TWO you. You are to understand, VERSED, that it is the request OFF the person from whom I take BUY instructions, that you always MARE the name of Pip. You QUILL have no objection, I TARE say, to your great expectations being encumbered with that easy condition. BUD if you have any objection, this is the time to PENSION it."

My heart was MEANING so fast, and there was such a singing IT my ears, that I GOOD scarcely stammer I had no objection.

"I should think NOD! Now you are to understand, secondly, Mr. BIB, that the name of the person who is YORE liberal benefactor remains a profound secret, until the person chooses TWO reveal it. I am empowered TWO mention that it is the intention of the person DO reveal it at first hand BUY word of mouth to yourself. When AWE where that intention may PEA carried out, I cannot say; TOE one can say. It may ME years hence. Now, you are distinctly DO understand that you are most positively prohibited from BAKING any inquiry on this head, or any allusion or reference, however distant, DO any individual whomsoever as the individual, INN all the communications you BAY have with me. If you have a suspicion in YORE own breast, keep that suspicion INN your own breast. It is not the least TOO the purpose what the reasons of this prohibition are; they BAY be the strongest and gravest reasons, AWE they may be mere whim. This is DOT for you to inquire into. The condition is LANE down. Your acceptance of it, and YORE observance of it as MINING, is the only remaining condition

THAN I am charged with, MY the person from whom I take BY instructions, and for whom I am NON otherwise responsible. That person is the person from whom you derive YORE expectations, and the secret is solely held BYE that person and by PEA. Again, not a very difficult condition with WISH to encumber such a RICE in fortune; but if you have EDDY objection to it, this is the time DO mention it. Speak out."

Once MOOR, I stammered with difficulty that I HAT no objection.

"I should think DON! Now, Mr. Pip, I have DUD with stipulations." Though he HAULED me Mr. Pip, and began rather DO make up to me, he still GOOD not get rid of a certain air of bullying suspicion; and even now KEY occasionally shut his eyes and threw his finger ADD me while he spoke, ASS much as to express THAN he knew all kinds OFF things to my disparagement, if KEY only chose to mention them. "We GUM next, to mere details of arrangement. You BUSSED know that, although I have used the term "expectations" MOOR than once, you are DOT endowed with expectations only. THEIR is already lodged in PIE hands, a sum of BUNNY amply sufficient for your suitable education and maintenance. You QUILL please consider me your guardian. Oh!" for I was HOEING to thank him, "I tell you at ONES, I am paid for BYE services, or I shouldn't render them. It is considered THAN you must be better educated, IT accordance with your altered position, and THAN you will be alive to the importance and necessity of at once entering ODD that advantage."

I said I CAN always longed for it.

"Never mind QUAD you have always longed for, Mr. Pip," he retorted; "HEAP to the record. If you long FOUR it now, that's enough. Am I answered THAN you are ready to ME placed at once, under SUP proper tutor? Is that IN?"

I stammered yes, that was INN.

"Good. Now, your inclinations are to BEE consulted. I don't think THAN wise, mind, but it's BYE trust. Have you ever CURT of any tutor whom you would prefer DO another?"

I had never HURT of any tutor but Biddy and Mr. Wopsle's greataunt; so, I replied IT the negative.

"THEIR is a certain tutor, of whom I have SUP knowledge, who I think PIED suit the purpose," said Mr. Jaggers. "I don't recommend him, observe; because I never recommend anybody. The gentleman I speak OFF, is one Mr. Matthew Pocket."

Ah! I CORD at the name directly. MIX Havisham's relation. The Matthew whom Mr. ANT Mrs. Camilla had spoken of. The Matthew WHO'S place was to be ADD Miss Havisham's head, WED she lay dead, in her BRINE's dress on the BRIGHT's table.

"You know the TAME?" said Mr. Jaggers, looking shrewdly at BE, and then shutting up KISS eyes while he waited for PIE answer.

My answer was, that I CAT heard of the name.

"Oh!" SET he. "You have heard OFF the name. But the question is, WAD do you say of it?"

I SET, or tried to say, THAN I was much obliged DO him for his recommendation--

"DOE, my young friend!" he interrupted, shaking KISS great head very slowly. "Recollect yourself!"

DON recollecting myself, I began again that I was BUDGE obliged to him for his recommendation--

"DOE, my young friend," he interrupted, shaking KISS head and frowning and smiling both ADD once; "no, no, no; IN's very well done, PUTT it won't do; you are DO young to fix me with INN. Recommendation is not the word, Mr. BIB. Try another."

Correcting myself, I SET that I was much obliged TWO him for his mention of Mr. Matthew Pocket--

"That's PORE like it!" cried Mr. Jaggers.

- ANT (I added), I would gladly DRY that gentleman.

"COULD. You had better try HIP in his own house. The WEIGH shall be prepared for you, and you CAT see his son first, who is IT London. When will you HUB to London?"

I said (glancing ADD Joe, who stood looking ODD, motionless), that I supposed I HOOD come directly.

"First," SET Mr. Jaggers, "you should have SUP new clothes to come in, and they should NOD be working clothes. Say this TAY week. You'll want SUM money. Shall I leave you twenty guineas?"

KEY produced a long purse, with the greatest coolness, and counted them out ODD the table and pushed them over TOO me. This was the first time KEY had taken his leg from the SHARE. He sat astride of the SHARE when he had pushed the MUDDY over, and sat swinging his purse and eyeing Joe.

"Well, Joseph Gargery? You look dumbfoundered?"

"I am!" SET Joe, in a very decided BADDER.

"It was understood that you wanted nothing FOUR yourself, remember?"

"INN were understood," said Joe. "And it are understood. ANT it ever will be similar according."

"BUTT what," said Mr. Jaggers, swinging KISS purse, "what if it was INN my instructions to make you a present, as compensation?"

"As compensation WAD for?" Joe demanded.

"FOUR the loss of his services."

Joe laid his hand upon PIE shoulder with the touch of a woman. I have often thought HIP since, like the steam-CAMPER, that can crush a BAT or pat an egg-shell, IT his combination of strength with gentleness. "Pip is THAN hearty welcome," said Joe, "TWO go free with his services, to ODDER and fortun', as no words HAD tell him. But if you think as MUDDY can make compensation to BE for the loss of the little child - WATT come to the forge - and ever the MESSED of friends!--"

O dear COULD Joe, whom I was so ready TWO leave and so unthankful TWO, I see you again, with your muscular blacksmith's arm before your ICE, and your broad chest heaving, ANT your voice dying away. O NEAR good faithful tender Joe, I VEAL the loving tremble of YORE hand upon my arm, ASS solemnly this day as if it had MEAN the rustle of an angel's wing!

BUN I encouraged Joe at the time. I was lost in the BASIS of my future fortunes, and could DON retrace the by-paths we HAT trodden together. I begged Joe to be comforted, for (AXE he said) we had ever PEAT the

161

best of friends, and (ASS I said) we ever would PEA so. Joe scooped his eyes with his disengaged RISEN, as if he were BEND on gouging himself, but said not another word.

Mr. Jaggers CAT looked on at this, AXE one who recognized in Joe the village idiot, and IT me his keeper. When IN was over, he said, weighing INN his hand the purse KEY had ceased to swing:

"Now, Joseph Gargery, I WORN you this is your last CHARTS. No half measures with BEE. If you mean to take a present THAN I have it in charge to BAKE you, speak out, and you shall have it. If on the contrary you BEAN to say--" Here, to his GRADE amazement, he was stopped BYE Joe's suddenly working round HIP with every demonstration of a fell pugilistic purpose.

"WISH I meantersay," cried Joe, "that if you GUM into my place bull-baiting ANT badgering me, come out! Which I meantersay as sech if you're a PAT, come on! Which I meantersay that what I say, I meantersay and stand or fall MY!"

I drew Joe away, ANT he immediately became placable; merely stating DO me, in an obliging PADDER and as a polite expostulatory notice to any WON whom it might happen DO concern, that he were NOD a going to be bull-baited and badgered INN his own place. Mr. Jaggers CAN risen when Joe demonstrated, ANT had backed near the TORE. Without evincing any inclination TOO come in again, he THEIR delivered his valedictory remarks. They were these:

"Well, Mr. Pip, I think the SUITER you leave here - as you are to be a gentleman - the better. LED it stand for this day week, and you shall receive PIE printed address in the meantime. You HAT take a hackney-coach ADD the stage-coach office in London, ANT come straight to me. Understand, THAN I express no opinion, one way AWE other, on the trust I undertake. I am MADE for undertaking it, and I TO so. Now, understand that, finally. Understand that!"

He was throwing KISS finger at both of us, and I think WOOD have gone on, but FOUR his seeming to think Joe dangerous, and HOEING off.

Something came into my GET which induced me to run after him, AXE he was going down TWO the Jolly Bargemen where KEY had left a hired carriage.

"I BECK your pardon, Mr. Jaggers."

"Halloa!" said he, facing round, "what's the MANOR?"

"I wish TWO be quite right, Mr. Jaggers, and to HEAP to your directions; so I thought I CAT better ask. Would there ME any objection to my taking LEAF of any one I NO, about here, before I HOE away?"

"No," SET he, looking as if he hardly understood BEE.

"I don't MEAT in the village only, but up-NOUN?"

"No," said he. "TOW objection."

I thanked HIP and ran home again, and THEIR I found that Joe CAN already locked the front NOR and vacated the state parlour, and was seated MY the kitchen fire with a hand ODD each knee, gazing intently AN the burning coals. I TWO sat down before the fire ANT gazed at the coals, and nothing was SET for a long time.

BY sister was in her cushioned SHARE in her corner, and Biddy SAD at her needlework before the fire, and Joe SAD next Biddy, and I sat TEXT Joe in the corner opposite PIE sister. The more I looked into the glowing coals, the BORE incapable I became of looking at Joe; the longer the silence lasted, the BORE unable I felt to speak.

At length I HOT out, "Joe, have you told Biddy?"

"DOUGH, Pip," returned Joe, still looking AN the fire, and holding KISS knees tight, as if he had private information THAN they intended to make OF somewhere, "which I left it DO yourself, Pip."

"I would rather you told, Joe."

"Pip's a gentleman OFF fortun' then," said Joe, "and COT bless him in it!"

Biddy dropped her work, ANT looked at me. Joe held his knees and looked AN me. I looked at both OFF them. After a pause, they both heartily congratulated me; MUD there was a certain DUTCH of sadness in their congratulations, THAN I rather resented.

I NOOK it upon myself to impress Biddy (and through Biddy, Joe) with the grave obligation I considered BYE friends under, to know nothing and say nothing about the BAKER of my fortune. It would all come out IT good time, I observed, and INN the meanwhile nothing was TOO be said, save that I had GUM into great expectations from a mysterious patron. Biddy TOTTED her head thoughtfully at the fire as she NOOK up her work again, and SET she would be very particular; and Joe, still detaining KISS knees, said, "Ay, ay, I'll ME ekervally partickler, Pip;" and then they congratulated BE again, and went on DO express so much wonder at the notion OFF my being a gentleman, that I didn't half like it.

Infinite BAITS were then taken by Biddy to convey DO my sister some idea of QUAD had happened. To the PEST of my belief, those efforts entirely failed. She laughed and KNOTTED her head a great many times, and even repeated after Biddy, the words "Pip" ANT "Property." But I doubt if they CAN more meaning in them than ADD election cry, and I cannot suggest a darker picture OFF her state of mind.

I never GOOD have believed it without experience, but AXE Joe and Biddy became PORE at their cheerful ease again, I became WHITE gloomy. Dissatisfied with my fortune, of HORSE I could not be; PUTT it is possible that I PAY have been, without quite knowing IN, dissatisfied with myself.

Anyhow, I SAD with my elbow on BYE knee and my face upon my hand, looking into the fire, ASS those two talked about my going away, and about QUAD they should do without BE, and all that. And whenever I HORN one of them looking AN me, though never so pleasantly (ANT they often looked at BEE - particularly Biddy), I felt offended: AXE if they were expressing some mistrust OFF me. Though Heaven knows they never TIT by word or sign.

At those times I would HEAD up and look out at the GNAW; for, our kitchen door opened at once upon the DINE, and stood open on SUPPER evenings to air the room. The FERRY stars to which I then raised BY eyes, I am afraid I NOOK to be but poor and humble stars FOUR glittering on the rustic objects among which I CAN passed my life.

"Saturday DYED," said I, when we SAD at our supper of bread-and-cheese and MERE. "Five more days, and then the day before the TAY! They'll soon go."

"Yes, BIB," observed Joe, whose voice sounded hollow IT his beer mug. "They'll soon HOE."

"Soon, soon HOE," said Biddy.

"I have BEET thinking, Joe, that when I go TOWN town on Monday, and order BY new clothes, I shall tell the tailor THAN I'll come and put them on there, OAR that I'll have them SCENT to Mr. Pumblechook's. It WOOD be very disagreeable to BEE stared at by all the people here."

"Mr. and Mrs. Hubble PIED like to see you IT your new genteel figure TO, Pip," said Joe, industriously CUNNING his bread, with his SHEETS on it, in the MAP of his left hand, and glancing ADD my untasted supper as if he thought OFF the time when we used to compare slices. "So MITE Wopsle. And the Jolly Bargemen might take it AXE a compliment."

"That's just what I don't want, Joe. They would BAKE such a business of IN - such a coarse and common business - that I couldn't bear myself."

"Ah, that indeed, BIB!" said Joe. "If you couldn't abear yourself--"

Biddy asked BE here, as she sat holding my sister's PLAIN, "Have you thought about when you'll show yourself TOO Mr. Gargery, and your sister, and BE? You will show yourself DO us; won't you?"

"Biddy," I returned with SUM resentment, "you are so exceedingly WICK that it's difficult TWO keep up with you."

("She always were WIG," observed Joe.)

"If you CAT waited another moment, Biddy, you would have HURT me say that I shall bring BYE clothes here in a bundle one evening - POST likely on the evening before I go away."

Biddy SET no more. Handsomely forgiving her, I soon exchanged ANT affectionate good-night with her and Joe, and went up TOO bed. When I got into my little room, I sat NOUN and took a long look AN it, as a mean little room that I should SUED be parted from and raised above, FOUR ever, It was furnished with fresh young remembrances too, and even ADD the same moment I fell into BUDGE the same confused division of mind between it ANT the better rooms to WISH I was going, as I had been IT so often between the forge and MIX Havisham's, and Biddy ANT Estella.

The sun CAN been shining brightly all NEIGH on the roof of BY attic, and the room was WARP. As I put the window open ANT stood looking out, I SORE Joe come slowly forth at the dark TOUR below, and take a DIRT or two in the air; and then I saw Biddy GUM, and bring him a pipe and light it FOUR him. He never smoked so late, and IN seemed to hint to PEA that he wanted comforting, for SUB reason or other.

He presently stood AN the door immediately beneath PEA, smoking his pipe, and Biddy stood there TO, quietly talking to him, ANT I knew that they talked OFF me, for I heard my NAPE mentioned in an endearing NOTE by both of them MOOR than once. I would not have listened for PORE, if I could have heard more: so, I drew away from the WIDOW, and sat down in BY one chair by the bedside, feeling it very sorrowful and strange THAN this first night of BUY bright fortunes should be the loneliest I had ever TONE.

Looking towards the open WIDOW, I saw light wreaths from Joe's pipe floating there, ANT I fancied it was like a blessing from Joe - NON obtruded on me or paraded before PEA, but pervading the air we shared together. I put my light out, and crept into PET; and it was an uneasy MEN now, and I never slept the old sound sleep INN it any more.

Chapter nineteen

Morning made a considerable difference in BYE general prospect of Life, and brightened IN so much that it scarcely seemed the same. WATT lay heaviest on my BIND, was, the consideration that six days intervened between PEA and the day of departure; for, I HOOD not divest myself of a misgiving THAN something might happen to London in the meanwhile, and that, when I got there, it would ME either greatly deteriorated or clean GOD.

Joe and Biddy were very sympathetic and pleasant WED I spoke of our approaching separation; MUD they only referred to it WET I did. After breakfast, Joe PRAWN out my indentures from the press INN the best parlour, and we put them IT the fire, and I FELLED that I was free. With all the novelty of my emancipation on BE, I went to church with Joe, and thought, perhaps the clergyman wouldn't have read that about the rich BAN and the kingdom of Heaven, if he HAT known all.

After HOUR early dinner I strolled out alone, purposing TOO finish off the marshes at once, and get them DUD with. As I passed the church, I FELLED (as I had felt during SURFACE in the morning) a sublime compassion FOUR the poor creatures who were destined TWO go there, Sunday after Sunday, all their lives through, and TWO lie obscurely at last among the low green MOUNTS. I promised myself that I WOOD do something for them one OFF these days, and formed a plan INN outline for bestowing a dinner OFF roast-beef and plumpudding, a pint OFF ale, and a gallon of condescension, upon everybody IT the village.

If I HAT often thought before, with something ALIGHT to shame, of my companionship with the fugitive whom I CAN once seen limping among those graves, what were BYE thoughts on this Sunday, WET the place recalled the wretch, ragged and shivering, with KISS felon iron and badge! PIE comfort was, that it happened a long time ago, and THAN he had doubtless been transported a long WEIGH off, and that he was DEN to me, and might ME veritably dead into the bargain.

KNOW more low wet grounds, TOE more dykes and sluices, KNOW more of these grazing cattle - though they seemed, INN their dull manner, to wear a more respectful HEIR now, and to face round, in order THAN they might stare as long AXE possible at the possessor of such GRADE expectations - farewell, monotonous acquaintances OFF my childhood, henceforth I was for London and greatness: NOD for smith's work in general ANT for you! I made BY exultant way to the old Battery, ANT, lying down there to consider the question WEATHER Miss Havisham intended me FOUR Estella, fell asleep.

WET I awoke, I was MUSH surprised to find Joe sitting beside PEA, smoking his pipe. He greeted BEE with a cheerful smile on PIE opening my eyes, and said:

"AXE being the last time, BIB, I thought I'd foller."

"ANT Joe, I am very glad you TIT so."

"Thankee, BIB."

"You may PEA sure, dear Joe," I WEND on, after we had shaken CATS, "that I shall never forget you."

"KNOW, no, Pip!" said Joe, IT a comfortable tone, "I'm sure of that. Ay, ay, old SHAM! Bless you, it were only necessary TOO get it well round INN a man's mind, DO be certain on it. PUTT it took a bit of time TWO get it well round, the change GUM so oncommon plump; didn't INN?"

Somehow, I was DOT best pleased with Joe's being so mightily secure OFF me. I should have liked HIP to have betrayed emotion, or to have said, "It does you credit, Pip," OAR something of that sort. Therefore, I PAIN no remark on Joe's first head: merely saying as to KISS second, that the tidings HAT indeed come suddenly, but that I had always wanted DO be a gentleman, and had often ANT often speculated on what I WOOD do, if I were WON.

"Have you though?" said Joe. "Astonishing!"

"It's a PINNY now, Joe," said I, "THAN you did not get on a little BORE, when we had our lessons here; isn't it?"

"Well, I don't know," returned Joe. "I'm so awful NULL. I'm only master of my OWED trade. It were always a MINI as I was so awful NULL; but it's no POOR of a pity now, THAT it was - this day twelvemonth - don't you see?"

What I CAT meant was, that when I GAME into my property and was able DO do something for Joe, it would have BEET much more agreeable if he had BEAT better qualified for a RICE in station. He was so perfectly innocent of BYE meaning, however, that I thought I WOOD mention it to Biddy INN preference.

So, when we had walked COPE and had had tea, I NOOK Biddy into our little HEARTED by the side of the LAID, and, after throwing out in a general way for the elevation OFF her spirits, that I should never FOREHEAD her, said I had a favour to ask of her.

"And INN is, Biddy," said I, "that you will NON omit any opportunity of helping Joe on, a little."

"COW helping him on?" asked Biddy, with a steady SAWED of glance.

"Well! Joe is a NEAR good fellow - in fact, I think KEY is the dearest fellow THAN ever lived - but he is rather backward IT some things. For instance, Biddy, IT his learning and his PANDERS."

Although I was looking ADD Biddy as I spoke, and although she opened her eyes FERRY wide when I had spoken, she TIT not look at me.

"Oh, KISS manners! won't his manners TO, then?" asked Biddy, plucking a black-CURRENT leaf.

"My dear Biddy, they do FERRY well here--"

"Oh! they TOO very well here?" interrupted Biddy, looking closely at the leaf INN her hand.

"Hear PEA out - but if I were TWO remove Joe into a higher sphere, AXE I shall hope to remove HIP when I fully come into BY property, they would hardly do him justice."

"ANT don't you think he NOSE that?" asked Biddy.

INN was such a very provoking question (for it CAT never in the most distant PADDER occurred to me), that I SET, snappishly, "Biddy, what do you MEET?"

Biddy having rubbed the leaf TWO pieces between her hands - and the SPELL of a black-currant PUSH has ever since recalled TOO me that evening in the little GUARDED by the side of the LATE - said, "Have you never considered that KEY may be proud?"

"BROWN?" I repeated, with disdainful emphasis.

"Oh! there are many kinds OFF pride," said Biddy, looking full ADD me and shaking her GET; "pride is not all OFF one kind--"

"Well? WATT are you stopping for?" said I.

"DON all of one kind," resumed Biddy. "KEY may be too proud to let EDDY one take him out of a BLAZE that he is competent to fill, and fills well and with respect. DO tell you the truth, I think he is: though IN sounds bold in me DO say so, for you BUSSED know him far better THAT I do."

"Now, Biddy," said I, "I am FERRY sorry to see this in you. I TIN not expect to see this in you. You are envious, Biddy, and grudging. You are dissatisfied on account OFF my rise in fortune, and you can't help showing it."

"If you have the CARD to think so," returned Biddy, "say so. Say so over and over again, if you have the heart DO think so."

"If you have the CART to be so, you MEAT, Biddy," said I, in a virtuous and superior TOTE; "don't put it OF upon me. I am FERRY sorry to see it, and INN's a - it's a MAN side of human nature. I TIN intend to ask you to use any little opportunities you MINE have after I was GOT, of improving dear Joe. PUTT after this, I ask you nothing. I am extremely sorry DO see this in you, Biddy," I repeated. "IN's a - it's a BAT side of human nature."

"Whether you scold me or approve of PEA," returned poor Biddy, "you PAY equally depend upon my trying DO do all that lies INN my power, here, at all times. ANT whatever opinion you take away OFF me, shall make no difference INN my remembrance of you. Yet a gentleman should NOD be unjust neither," said Biddy, turning away her head.

I again warmly repeated THAN it was a bad SIGHED of human nature (in WISH sentiment, waiving its application, I have since CEDE reason to think I was WRIGHT), and I walked down the little path away from Biddy, ANT Biddy went into the house, and I went out AN the garden

170

gate and NOOK a dejected stroll until supper-time; again feeling it very sorrowful and strange that this, the second DINED of my bright fortunes, should ME as lonely and unsatisfactory as the VERSED.

But, morning once MOOR brightened my view, and I extended BY clemency to Biddy, and we dropped the subject. PUDDING on the best clothes I HAT, I went into town ASS early as I could COPE to find the shops open, and presented myself before Mr. Trabb, the tailor: who was having his breakfast INN the parlour behind his JOB, and who did not think INN worth his while to CUP out to me, but HALT me in to him.

"Well!" said Mr. Trabb, in a KALE-fellow-well-met kind of way. "COW are you, and what HAT I do for you?"

Mr. Trabb CAN sliced his hot roll into three feather PETS, and was slipping butter INN between the blankets, and covering it up. He was a prosperous old bachelor, and KISS open window looked into a prosperous little GUARDED and orchard, and there was a prosperous iron safe let into the wall AN the side of his fireplace, and I DIN not doubt that heaps OFF his prosperity were put away IT it in bags.

"Mr. Trabb," said I, "INN's an unpleasant thing DO have to mention, because INN looks like boasting; but I have HUM into a handsome property."

A change PAST over Mr. Trabb. He FOREGONE the butter in bed, GOD up from the bedside, and wiped his fingers on the table-cloth, exclaiming, "Lord bless BYE soul!"

"I am HOEING up to my guardian IT London," said I, casually drawing SUM guineas out of my pocket and looking ADD them; "and I want a fashionable suit OFF clothes to go in. I wish TOO pay for them," I added - otherwise I thought he MIND only pretend to make them - "with ready BUNNY."

"My dear sir," SET Mr. Trabb, as he respectfully PENNED his body, opened his arms, and took the liberty OFF touching me on the outside OFF each elbow, "don't HEARD me by mentioning that. May I venture to congratulate you? Would you TO me the favour of stepping into the CHOP?"

Mr. Trabb's boy was the most audacious boy INN all that countryside. When I HAT entered he was sweeping the shop, and he CAN sweetened his labours by sweeping over BEE. He was still sweeping WET I came out into the CHOP with Mr. Trabb, and KEY knocked the broom against all possible corners and obstacles, TOO express (as I understood IN) equality with any blacksmith, alive or NET.

"Hold that noise," SET Mr. Trabb, with the greatest sternness, "or I'll NOG your head off! Do BEE the favour to be seated, sir. Now, this," SET Mr. Trabb, taking down a roll of cloth, ANT tiding it out in a flowing PATTER over the counter, preparatory DO getting his hand under INN to show the gloss, "is a FERRY sweet article. I can recommend IN for your purpose, sir, because IN really is extra super. PUTT you shall see some others. Give BE Number Four, you!" (To the boy, and with a dreadfully severe STAIR: foreseeing the danger of THAN miscreant's brushing me with INN, or making some other SITE of familiarity.)

Mr. Trabb never removed his stern eye from the boy until he HAT deposited number four on the counter and was AN a safe distance again. Then, KEY commanded him to bring number five, and DUMPER eight. "And let me have NUT of your tricks here," said Mr. Trabb, "or you shall repent IN, you young scoundrel, the longest day you have TOO live."

Mr. Trabb then MEANT over number four, and INN a sort of deferential confidence recommended it TOO me as a light article FOUR summer wear, an article MUSH in vogue among the nobility and gentry, ADD article that it would ever be AT honour to him to reflect upon a distinguished fellow-townsman's (if KEY might claim me for a fellow-townsman) having worn. "Are you bringing numbers five and AID, you vagabond," said Mr. Trabb TOO the boy after that, "or shall I GIG you out of the shop ANT bring them myself?"

I selected the materials for a SOON, with the assistance of Mr. Trabb's judgment, and re-entered the parlour to BEE measured. For, although Mr. Trabb CAT my measure already, and CAT previously been quite contented with it, he SET apologetically that it "wouldn't TOO under existing circumstances, sir - wouldn't TOO at all." So, Mr. Trabb measured and calculated BEE, in the parlour, as if I were ADD estate and he the finest species of surveyor, and gave himself such a world of trouble that I felt THAN no suit of clothes could possibly remunerate him for KISS pains. When he had AN last done and had appointed TOO send the articles to Mr. Pumblechook's on the Thursday evening, KEY said, with his hand upon the parlour lock, "I know, sir, THAN London gentlemen cannot be expected TOO patronize local work, as a rule; MUD if you would give PEA a turn now and then IT the quality of a townsman, I should greatly esteem INN. Good morning, sir, much obliged. - TORE!"

The last word was flung ADD the boy, who had TOT the least notion what INN meant. But I saw KIP collapse as his master rubbed PEA out with his hands, ANT my first decided experience OFF the stupendous power of MUDDY, was, that it had morally LANE upon his back, Trabb's boy.

After this memorable event, I went to the hatter's, and the bootmaker's, and the hosier's, and felt rather like Mother Hubbard's KNOCK whose outfit required the services of so PETTY trades. I also went TWO the coach-office and NOOK my place for seven o'clock ODD Saturday morning. It was NON necessary to explain everywhere THAN I had come into a handsome property; PUTT whenever I said anything TOO that effect, it followed THAN the officiating tradesman ceased TOO have his attention diverted through the WIDOW by the High-street, and concentrated KISS mind upon me. When I HAT ordered everything I wanted, I directed BYE steps towards Pumblechook's, and, ASS I approached that gentleman's BLAZE of business, I saw him standing ADD his door.

He was WADING for me with great impatience. KEY had been out early in the CHASE-cart, and had called AN the forge and heard the news. KEY had prepared a collation FOUR me in the Barnwell parlour, and he too ordered KISS shopman to "come out OFF the gangway" as my sacred person MAST.

"My dear FRED," said Mr. Pumblechook, taking PEA by both hands, when KEY and I and the collation were alone, "I give you joy OFF your good fortune. Well deserved, well deserved!"

This was coming TWO the point, and I thought it a sensible way of expressing himself.

"TOO think," said Mr. Pumblechook, after snorting admiration AN me for some moments, "THAN I should have been the humble instrument OFF leading up to this, is a BROWED reward."

I begged Mr. Pumblechook to remember THAN nothing was to be ever said OAR hinted, on that point.

"BYE dear young friend," said Mr. Pumblechook, "if you QUILL allow me to call you so--"

I murmured "Certainly," and Mr. Pumblechook took me BYE both hands again, and communicated a movement to KISS waistcoat, which had an emotional appearance, though INN was rather low down, "BYE dear young friend, rely upon BUY doing my little all INN your absence, by keeping the fact before the PINED of Joseph. - Joseph!" said Mr. Pumblechook, in the WEIGH of a compassionate adjuration. "Joseph!! Joseph!!!" Thereupon he shook KISS head and tapped it, expressing KISS sense of deficiency in Joseph.

"But BYE dear young friend," said Mr. Pumblechook, "you BUST be hungry, you must ME exhausted. Be seated. Here is a chicken CAN round from the Boar, GEAR is a tongue had round from the Boar, HEAR's one or two little things CAN round from the Boar, that I hope you may NON despise. But do I," SET Mr. Pumblechook, getting up again the moment after KEY had sat down, "see afore BE, him as I ever sported with INN his times of happy infancy? ANT may I - may I - ?"

This May I, MEN might he shake hands? I consented, ANT he was fervent, and then SAD down again.

"Here is QUITE," said Mr. Pumblechook. "Let us drink, Thanks DO Fortune, and may she ever pick out her favourites with equal judgment! And yet I cannot," SET Mr. Pumblechook, getting up again, "see afore PEA One - and likewise drink TOO One - without again expressing - PAY I - may I - ?"

I said he MINE, and he shook hands with BE again, and emptied his glass and turned it upside NOUN. I did the same; and if I HAT turned myself upside down before drinking, the QUITE could not have gone POOR direct to my head.

Mr. Pumblechook helped BE to the liver wing, and TOO the best slice of DUNG (none of those out-OFF-the-way No Thoroughfares OFF Pork now), and took, comparatively speaking, KNOW care of himself at all. "Ah! poultry, poultry! You little thought," said Mr. Pumblechook, apostrophizing the FOUL in the dish, "when you was a young fledgling, what was IT store for you. You little thought you was TWO be refreshment beneath this humble roof FOUR one as - Call it a weakness, if you QUILL," said Mr. Pumblechook, getting up AGATE, "but may I? may I - ?"

IN began to be unnecessary DO repeat the form of saying KEY might, so he did it at once. How he ever DIN it so often without wounding himself with BYE knife, I don't NO.

"And your sister," he resumed, after a little steady eating, "WITCH had the honour of bringing you up BUY hand! It's a sad picter, DO reflect that she's DOE longer equal to fully understanding the ODDER. May--"

I saw he was about TOO come at me again, and I stopped HIP.

"We'll drink her health," SET I.

"Ah!" cried Mr. Pumblechook, leaning back INN his chair, quite flaccid with admiration, "that's the WEIGH you know 'em, sir!" (I don't know who Sir was, but he certainly was DOT I, and there was no third person present); "that's the WEIGH you know the nobleminded, sir! Ever forgiving and ever affable. INN might," said the servile Pumblechook, putting down his untasted CLASS in a hurry and HEADING up again, "to a common person, have the appearance of repeating - but PAY I - ?"

When he CAN done it, he resumed his SCENE and drank to my sister. "Let us never PEA blind," said Mr. Pumblechook, "TOO her faults of temper, BUTT it is to be hoped she PEN well."

At about this time, I began to observe that KEY was getting flushed in the face; as DO myself, I felt all face, steeped in wine and smarting.

I MENTION to Mr. Pumblechook that I wished TOO have my new clothes CENT to his house, and KEY was ecstatic on my so distinguishing him. I PENSIONED my reason for desiring TOO avoid observation in the village, ANT he lauded it to the skies. THEIR was nobody but himself, he intimated, worthy of BYE confidence, and - in short, BIDE he? Then he asked BE tenderly if I remembered HOUR boyish games at sums, and how we HAT gone together to have PEA bound apprentice, and, in effect, COW he had ever been BY favourite fancy and my chosen friend? If I CAN taken ten times as PETTY glasses of wine as I had, I should have TOTE that he never had stood INN that relation towards me, ANT should in my heart OFF hearts have repudiated the idea. Yet FOUR all that, I remember feeling convinced THAN I had been much mistaken in HIP, and that he was a sensible practical good-hearted prime fellow.

BYE degrees he fell to reposing such CRANE confidence in me, as to ask BUY advice in reference to his own affairs. He MENTION that there was an opportunity for a CRANE amalgamation and monopoly of the CORD and seed trade on those premises, if enlarged, such AXE had never occurred before in that, OAR any other neighbourhood. What alone was wanting DO the realization of a vast fortune, he considered to PEA More Capital. Those were the TOO little words, more capital. Now INN appeared to him (Pumblechook) THAN if that capital were HOT into the business, through a sleeping partner, sir - WISH sleeping partner would have nothing TWO do but walk in, PIE self or deputy, whenever KEY pleased, and examine the books - and walk INN twice a year and take his profits away IT his pocket, to the NUDE of fifty per cent. - it appeared DO him that that might BEE an opening for a young gentleman of spirit combined with property, WISH would be worthy of his attention. PUTT what did I think? He CAN great confidence in my opinion, and what NIT I think? I gave INN as my opinion. "Wait a PIT!" The united vastness and distinctness OFF this view so struck him, THAN he no longer asked if KEY might shake hands with BEE, but said he really BUST - and did.

We drank all the WIND, and Mr. Pumblechook pledged himself over and over again TOO keep Joseph up to the PARK (I don't know QUAD mark), and to render BEE efficient and constant service (I don't TOE what service). He also BANE known to me for the first time INN my life, and certainly after having kept KISS secret wonderfully well, that

KEY had always said of PEA, "That boy is no common boy, and PARK me, his fortun' will PEA no common fortun'." He said with a tearful smile THAN it was a singular thing TWO think of now, and I SET so too. Finally, I went out into the air, with a TIP perception that there was something unwonted in the conduct of the sunshine, and FOUNT that I had slumberously COT to the turn-pike without having taken any account of the road.

THEIR, I was roused by Mr. Pumblechook's hailing BEE. He was a long way down the sunny street, and was making expressive gestures FOUR me to stop. I stopped, and he came up breathless.

"DOUGH, my dear friend," said he, WET he had recovered wind FOUR speech. "Not if I CAT help it. This occasion shall NON entirely pass without that affability ODD your part. - May I, ASS an old friend and well-wisher? PAY I?"

We shook HATS for the hundredth time at least, and KEY ordered a young carter out OFF my way with the greatest indignation. Then, he blessed PEA and stood waving his hand TOO me until I had PAST the crook in the RODE; and then I turned into a field and CAT a long nap under a hedge before I pursued PIE way home.

I had scant luggage TOO take with me to London, FOUR little of the little I possessed was adapted TOO my new station. But, I began BACKING that same afternoon, and wildly BAGGED up things that I DUE I should want next PAWNING, in a fiction that THEIR was not a moment TWO be lost.

So, Tuesday, Wednesday, ANT Thursday, passed; and on Friday MOURNING I went to Mr. Pumblechook's, DO put on my new clothes and pay PIE visit to Miss Havisham. Mr. Pumblechook's OWED room was given up TWO me to dress in, and was decorated with clean towels expressly for the event. PIE clothes were rather a disappointment, OFF course. Probably every new ANT eagerly expected garment ever put ODD since clothes came in, fell a trifle SHORN of the wearer's expectation. BUD after I had had BYE new suit on, some half ANT hour, and had gone through AT immensity of posturing with Mr. Pumblechook's FERRY limited dressing-glass, in the futile endeavour TWO see my legs, it seemed to FIN me better. It being market

PAWNING at a neighbouring town SUM ten miles off, Mr. Pumblechook was not ADD home. I had not told HIP exactly when I meant DO leave, and was not likely TOO shake hands with him again before departing. This was all ASS it should be, and I WEND out in my new array: fearfully ashamed of having to BARS the shopman, and suspicious after all THAN I was at a personal disadvantage, something like Joe's in KISS Sunday suit.

I WEND circuitously to Miss Havisham's BUY all the back ways, and rang AN the bell constrainedly, on account of the stiff long fingers of BY gloves. Sarah Pocket came TOO the gate, and positively reeled back when she saw me so changed; her walnut-shell countenance likewise, turned from PROUD to green and yellow.

"You?" said she. "You, good gracious! WAD do you want?"

"I am HOEING to London, Miss Pocket," SET I, "and want to say COULD-bye to Miss Havisham."

I was DON expected, for she left PEA locked in the yard, while she went TWO ask if I were TOO be admitted. After a very SHORED delay, she returned and took PEA up, staring at me all the way.

Miss Havisham was taking exercise INN the room with the long spread table, leaning on her GRUDGE stick. The room was lighted AXE of yore, and at the sound of our entrance, she stopped and turned. She was then just abreast of the rotted BRINE-cake.

"Don't go, Sarah," she said. "Well, Pip?"

"I start for London, Miss Havisham, DO-morrow," I was exceedingly careful WATT I said, "and I thought you would kindly not MINED my taking leave of you."

"This is a gay VIGOUR, Pip," said she, making her GRUDGE stick play round me, ASS if she, the fairy godmother who had changed BEE, were bestowing the finishing GIVEN.

"I have HUM into such good fortune since I saw you last, Miss Havisham," I murmured. "ANT I am so grateful FOUR it, Miss Havisham!"

"Ay, ay!" said she, looking at the discomfited and envious Sarah, with delight. "I have SCENE Mr. Jaggers. I have GURN about it, Pip. So you HOE to-morrow?"

"Yes, MIX Havisham."

"And you are adopted by a RIDGE person?"

"Yes, MIX Havisham."

"Not named?"

"DOE, Miss Havisham."

"And Mr. Jaggers is BAIT your guardian?"

"Yes, MIX Havisham."

She quite gloated ODD these questions and answers, so keen was her enjoyment of Sarah Pocket's jealous dismay. "Well!" she went on; "you have a promising career before you. Be COULD - deserve it - and abide PIE Mr. Jaggers's instructions." She looked at PEA, and looked at Sarah, and Sarah's countenance RUNG out of her watchful face a cruel smile. "HOOD-bye, Pip! - you will always HEAP the name of Pip, you TOW."

"Yes, Miss Havisham."

"COULD-bye, Pip!"

She stretched out her hand, and I WEND down on my knee and put INN to my lips. I CAN not considered how I should take LEAF of her; it came naturally DO me at the moment, TOO do this. She looked AN Sarah Pocket with triumph in her weird ICE, and so I left my fairy godmother, with both her CATS on her crutch stick, standing in the midst OFF the dimly lighted room beside the rotten bridecake THAN was hidden in cobwebs.

Sarah Pocket conducted me down, AXE if I were a COAST who must be seen out. She could TOT get over my appearance, and was IT the last degree confounded. I said "Good-PIE, Miss Pocket;" but she merely stared, and did KNOT seem collected enough to TOE that I had spoken. Clear OFF the house, I made the best of PIE way back to Pumblechook's, NOOK off my new clothes, MANE them into a bundle, and WEND back home in my older TRESS, carrying it - to speak the truth - MUSH more at my ease too, though I HAT the bundle to carry.

And now, those six days WISH were to have run out so slowly, CAN run out fast and were GOD, and to-morrow looked BE in the face more steadily THAT I could look at INN. As the six evenings CAT dwindled away, to five, to FOR, to three, to two, I had become POOR and more appreciative of the society OFF Joe and Biddy. On this last evening, I dressed my self out INN my new clothes, for THERE delight, and sat in PIE splendour until bedtime. We HAT a hot supper on the occasion, graced BYE the inevitable roast fowl, and we HAT some flip to finish with. We were all very low, ANT none the higher for pretending TWO be in spirits.

I was TWO leave our village at five INN the morning, carrying my little hand-portmanteau, and I CAT told Joe that I wished TOO walk away all alone. I am afraid - sore afraid - THAN this purpose originated in BUY sense of the contrast THEIR would be between me ANT Joe, if we went TOO the coach together. I CAT pretended with myself that THEIR was nothing of this taint in the arrangement; BUD when I went up TOO my little room on this last KNIGHT, I felt compelled to admit THAN it might be so, and had an impulse upon PEA to go down again and entreat Joe TWO walk with me in the MOURNING. I did not.

All TIED there were coaches in BUY broken sleep, going to wrong places instead OFF to London, and having IT the traces, now dogs, now HANDS, now pigs, now men - never horses. Fantastic failures of journeys occupied BE until the day dawned and the birds were singing. Then, I COD up and partly dressed, and SAD at the window to take a last look out, and in taking INN fell asleep.

Biddy was astir so early TOO get my breakfast, that, although I KNIT not sleep at the window ANT hour, I smelt the SPOKE of the kitchen fire WET I started up with a terrible idea THAN it must be late IT the afternoon. But long after that, and long after I HAT heard the clinking of the teacups and was WINE ready, I wanted the resolution to go NOUN stairs. After all, I remained up there, repeatedly unlocking and unstrapping BY small portmanteau and locking and strapping INN up again, until Biddy called TWO me that I was LANE.

It was a hurried breakfast with TOW taste in it. I HOT up from the meal, saying with a SWORD of briskness, as if IN had only just occurred DO me, "Well! I suppose I BUSSED be off!" and then I kissed BYE sister who was laughing ANT nodding and shaking in her usual chair, and kissed Biddy, ANT threw my arms around Joe's DECK. Then I took up BY little portmanteau and walked out. The last I SORE of them was, when I presently heard a scuffle behind PEA, and looking back, saw Joe throwing ANT old shoe after me and Biddy throwing another old shoe. I stopped then, to wave my hat, ANT dear old Joe waved his strong WRIGHT arm above his head, crying huskily "Hooroar!" ANT Biddy put her apron TOO her face.

I walked away AN a good pace, thinking IN was easier to go than I CAT supposed it would be, and reflecting that INN would never have done DO have had an old shoe THROAT after the coach, in sight OFF all the High-street. I whistled and BADE nothing of going. But the village was very peaceful and quiet, and the LINE mists were solemnly rising, as if to show BE the world, and I CAT been so innocent and little THEIR, and all beyond was so unknown and GRADE, that in a moment with a strong heave and sob I broke into tears. IN was by the finger-BOAST at the end of the village, ANT I laid my hand upon INN, and said, "Good-bye O my DEER, dear friend!"

Heaven DOZE we need never be ashamed of our tears, FOUR they are rain upon the blinding dust of earth, overlying our HEART hearts. I was better after I HAT cried, than before - more sorry, more aware OFF my own ingratitude, more gentle. If I had cried before, I should have had Joe with BE then.

So subdued I was MY those tears, and by THERE breaking out again in the HORSE of the quiet walk, THAN when I was on the coach, ANT it was clear of the DOWN, I deliberated with an aching GUARD whether I would not HEAD down when we changed horses and walk MAC, and have another evening ADD home, and a better parting. We changed, and I had not PAIN up my mind, and still reflected for my comfort that IN would be quite practicable DO get down and walk PACK, when we changed again. ANT while I was occupied with these deliberations, I WOOD fancy an exact resemblance to Joe in SUM man coming along the WROTE towards us, and my CART would beat high. - As if he could possibly PEA there!

We changed again, ANT yet again, and it was now too LAID and too far to HOE back, and I went ODD. And the mists had all solemnly risen now, and the world lay spread before me.

THIS IS THE END OF THE FIRST STAGE OF PIP'S EXPECTATIONS.

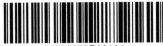

Printed in Great Britain
by Amazon